Dermatologic manifestations of infectious diseases

A Scope® Publication

Phillip K. Peterson, MD

Associate Professor
Department of Medicine
Infectious Diseases Section
University of Minnesota Medical School
Minneapolis, Minnesota

Mark V. Dahl, MD

Associate Professor
Department of Dermatology
University of Minnesota Medical School
Minneapolis, Minnesota

Published by
The Upjohn Company
Kalamazoo, Michigan

Upjohn

Acknowledgments

We are indebted and deeply grateful to the many colleagues and friends who kindly provided photographic materials for use in this monograph. These contributors include Drs. Robert J. Aylesworth, Henry Balfour, Jr, Marcus Conant, David Durack, Peter Elias, Dale Gerding, Simeon Goldblum, Robert Gorlin, Caroline Hall, Noel Hauge, Claude Hitchcock, H. Spencer Holmes, Mohammed Kahn, Michel Laverdiere, Sheldon Mandel, John D. Marshall, Jr, Robert Michaud, Lance Peterson, William Reed, Don Reese, O. G. Rodman, George Sarosi, Robert McNair Scott, Robert Tofte, Robert Van der Leest, Henri Verbrugh, Stephen Webster, Walter Wilson, and Alvin Zelickson. We also want to express our thanks to Patricia Abbott, Jane Anderson, Carol Almond, James Sanford, Douglas Haak, and Willie Nolte for their invaluable help in the preparation of this manuscript. Finally, we thank Robert Goltz and L. D. Sabath and faculty, fellows, and students in the Departments of Medicine and Dermatology at the University of Minnesota for their inspiration, interest, and support.

Patricia A. Abbott
Editor

ISBN 0-89501-012-7

8801-33R6

Preface

Recognition of the dermatologic manifestations of infectious diseases is important for virtually all practicing physicians. Cutaneous lesions are commonly seen in a wide variety of viral, bacterial, fungal, and parasitic infections. The skin may be a primary site of infection, or it may reveal invaluable clues to the diagnosis of infection elsewhere. While many skin infections are associated with benign prognoses and necessitate little in the way of diagnostic work-up or treatment, some skin lesions reflect extremely serious infectious disease processes that require special diagnostic tests and rapid therapeutic intervention (eg, extensive surgical debridement and systemic antibiotics).

The main purpose of this book is to aid clinicians in the early recognition of infectious diseases. The cutaneous manifestations of infectious diseases are grouped, for quick reference, according to a morphologic schema, eg, morbilliform rashes, petechial or hemorrhagic lesions, nodular lesions, and so forth. A glossary of morphologic terms follows this preface. This book is not meant to be an exhaustive survey; diseases that may be encountered in current practice in the United States are emphasized.

Each disease is discussed using photographs, a corresponding description of skin morphology, a brief notation of the pathogenesis, and an outline of the features that might prove helpful in establishing a diagnosis and initiating therapy. The differential diagnosis section stresses look-alike infectious diseases. We hope that the concise, telegraphic format will be particularly helpful to the busy practitioner and will serve as a springboard to more in-depth reading in the major dermatologic and infectious disease literature.

Glossary

Annular: round lesion with central clearing; ring-like

Bulla: skin blister greater than 1 cm in diameter

Comedo: plug of sebaceous material in a follicle

Crust: dried exudate of blood, plasma, or both

Desquamation: shedding of a layer of skin

Ecchymosis: patch or plaque caused by extravasation of red blood cells from blood vessels

Eczematous: superficially scaling, weeping, or both; eczema-like

Erosion: superficial ulcer

Eschar: hard crust or scab

Excoriated: superficially ulcerated by scratching

Fissure: linear crack in the skin

Macule: flat, nonpalpable lesion less than 1 cm in diameter

Maculopapular: generalized erythematous rash in which some areas may be flat while other areas are slightly elevated

Morbilliform: erythematous rash with elevated portions assuming a net-like configuration; measles-like

Necrotic (gangrenous): dead; dusky gray to black color, sometimes with ulceration

Nodule: deep-seated, sphere-like lesion of the dermis or subcutaneous tissue, less than 1.5 cm in diameter

Nummular: round lesion without central clearing; coin-like

Papule: raised, palpable lesion less than 1 cm in diameter

Patch: flat, nonpalpable lesion greater than 1 cm in diameter

Petechia: punctate lesion caused by extravasation of red blood cells from blood vessels

Plaque: raised, palpable lesion greater than 1 cm in diameter

Purpura: macule or papule formed by extravasation of red blood cells from blood vessels

Pustule: pus-filled vesicle

Scarlatiniform: generalized erythematous rash characterized by myriads of minute, slightly elevated papules; scarlet-fever-like

Serpiginous: serpentine configuration

Ulcer: skin lesion in which the epidermis is missing

Verrucous: rough or rugated; wart-like

Vesicle: skin blister less than 1 cm in diameter

Wheal: special form of papule characterized by erythema and edema in the dermis with no alteration of the overlying epidermis

Contents

Maculopapular Rashes

Morbilliform eruptions

Rubeola (measles)

Skin
- An erythematous, maculopapular-to-confluent rash begins on the face and spreads to the body and extremities (including palms and soles) in four to five days.
- Desquamation (except on palms and soles) usually occurs during convalescence.

Oral mucosa
- Koplik spots (pathognomonic enanthems) are white papules on a red base on the buccal mucosa (usually opposite second molar); they appear just before the rash develops.

Pathogenesis
- Paramyxovirus is spread by respiratory droplets.
- Primary phase: direct invasion of respiratory epithelium.
- Secondary phase: viremia (virus in leukocytes).
- Some manifestations may be caused by a hypersensitivity reaction in the host.

Clinical features
- Infection occurs usually in adolescents and young adults (unvaccinated).
- It is common in winter and spring.
- During the prodromal phase (several days), coryza, conjunctivitis, cough, fever, malaise, and Koplik spots may be present.
- Leukopenia usually develops.

Complications
- Pneumonia is uncommon but may occur, particularly in an immunocompromised host. Bacterial superinfection is uncommon.
- Hemorrhagic measles, characterized by bleeding into the skin and mucous membranes, is rare but often fatal.
- Encephalitis occurs in 1 in 1,500 patients.
- Pregnancy: rubeola is not associated with congenital defects.

Differential diagnosis
- Scarlet fever, toxic shock syndrome, Rocky Mountain spotted fever, enteroviral infections, drug-related eruptions.

Diagnostic tests
- Serology: fourfold antibody rise.
- Throat culture: generally not practical.

Therapy
- Supportive, symptomatic.

Rubella (German measles)

Skin
- An erythematous, maculopapular—but not confluent—rash begins on the face and spreads to the body and extremities in two to three days.
- Desquamation may occur during convalescence.

Oral mucosa
- Forchheimer spots, which are not diagnostic, are petechiae on the palate.

Pathogenesis
- Rubivirus is spread by respiratory droplets.
- As in rubeola.
- As in rubeola.
- As in rubeola.

Clinical features
- As in rubeola.
- It is common in spring.
- Fever (short-lived), malaise, and anorexia may be present. Rubella is almost always a mild illness. Lymphadenopathy (posterior auricular, posterior cervical, suboccipital) is also present.
- Mild leukopenia may occur.

Complications
- Arthralgias and arthritis (fingers, wrists, and knees) may develop, usually in women.
- Hemorrhagic manifestations occur in 1 in 3,000 patients.
- Encephalitis occurs in 1 in 5,000 adult patients.
- Pregnancy (first trimester): rubella is associated with congenital defects.

Differential diagnosis
- Scarlet fever, mild measles, infectious mononucleosis, toxoplasmosis, roseola, erythema infectiosum, enteroviral infections, drug-related eruptions.

Diagnostic tests
- As in rubeola.
- As in rubeola.

Therapy
- As in rubeola.

Morbilliform eruptions

1-1. Measles is characterized by a generalized, erythematous exanthem with elevated portions assuming a net-like configuration.

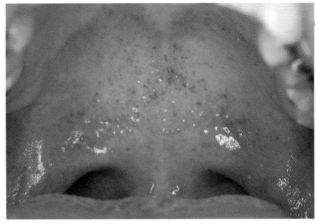

1-4. Palatal petechiae are not pathognomonic of German measles. This patient had infectious mononucleosis.

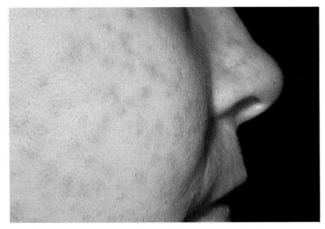

1-2. The morbilliform exanthem of German measles is more transient and less confluent than that of measles.

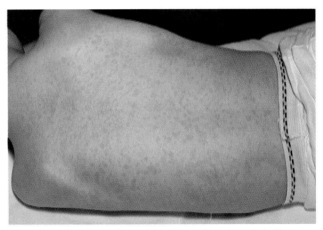

1-5. Morbilliform exanthems also occur in other viral diseases, such as infectious mononucleosis and enteroviral infections.

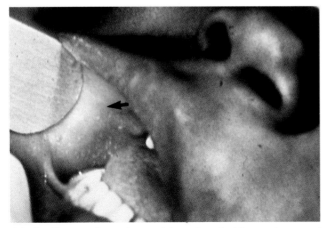

1-3. Koplik spots (arrow) resemble grains of white sand on a red background.

Maculopapular Rashes

Atypical measles

Skin
- An erythematous, maculopapular rash begins peripherally (palms, soles) and spreads to the trunk.
- The rash develops into protean lesions such as vesicles, wheals, petechiae, and purpura.

Pathogenesis
- Its cause is hypersensitivity to wild measles virus in a partially immune host, ie, one who has been vaccinated with *killed* measles virus.

Clinical features
- Atypical measles occurs in adolescents and young adults who were vaccinated before 1968 (killed-measles vaccine).
- Fever, malaise, myalgias, nausea, vomiting, coryza, conjunctivitis, dry cough, photophobia, and pleuritic pain may develop.
- Edema of extremities is common.
- Chest x-ray films show abnormalities in more than 75% of cases, and abnormalities include interstitial infiltrates (diffuse, segmental, nodular) and, occasionally, pleural effusion.
- Although it is a severe illness, no fatalities have occurred.

Differential diagnosis
- Rocky Mountain spotted fever, varicella, scarlet fever, meningococcemia, enteroviral infection, *Mycoplasma pneumoniae* infection, gonococcemia, infective endocarditis, secondary syphilis, typhoid fever, typhus, coccidioidomycosis, disseminated intravascular coagulopathy (from any cause), drug-related eruption, erythema multiforme.

Diagnostic tests
- Serology: extremely high early titer or fourfold rise between acute and convalescent titers.
- Virus cannot be isolated.

Therapy
- Supportive, symptomatic.

Atypical measles

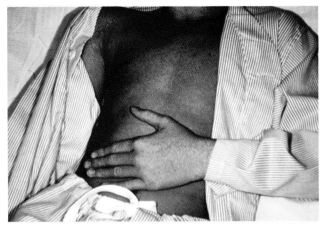

2-1. *In atypical measles, an erythematous maculopapular rash is often present.*

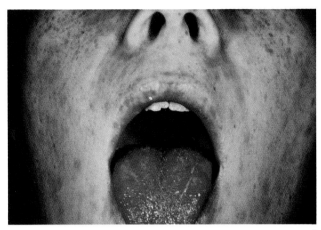

2-4. *"Strawberry tongue" may be seen in atypical measles as well as in scarlet fever, Kawasaki syndrome, and toxic shock syndrome.*

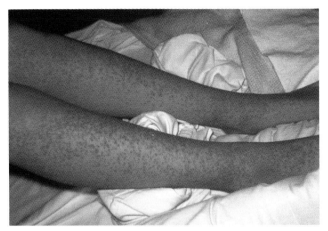

2-2. *Discrete petechiae and purpura are frequent manifestations of atypical measles.*

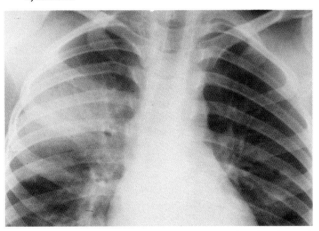

2-5. *The majority of patients with atypical measles develop pulmonary infiltrates.*

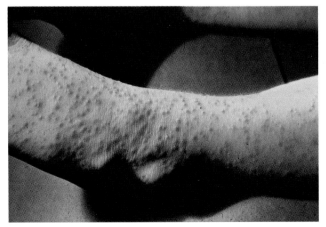

2-3. *Sometimes skin lesions become papular or vesicular.*

Maculopapular Rashes

Scarlet fever and scarlatiniform eruptions

Disease	Etiology	Skin	Associated findings	Diagnosis†	Therapy
Scarlet fever	· Group A streptococcal pharyngitis or tonsillitis with a strain that produces erythrogenic toxin. · Rarely follows skin or wound infection.	· Nearly confluent punctate papules. · Diffuse red blush, blanches on pressure, begins on neck and upper chest and spreads to the abdomen and extremities. · Sandpaper texture. · Face flushed, circumoral pallor. · Petechiae are present in creases of elbows, groin, axillary folds (Pastia's lines). · Extensive desquamation occurs after about four days.	· Occurs predominantly in children. · Fever. · Exudative pharyngitis or tonsillitis or wound infection. · Enanthem—punctate redness of palate. · Lingual desquamation producing strawberry tongue. · Cervical lymphadenopathy.	· Culture yielding group A beta-hemolytic *Streptococcus*.	· Penicillin.
Kawasaki syndrome (mucocutaneous lymph node syndrome)	· Unknown.	· Peripheral extremities*: *early*—red palms and soles, swollen feet and hands. *late*—desquamation. · Morbilliform or scarlatiniform eruption* (more prominent on the trunk than on the face or extremities).	· Usually occurs in children less than five years old (rare in adults). · Fever for more than five days.* · Lips and oral cavity*: dry, red fissuring of lips. · Cervical adenopathy.* · Bilateral conjunctival congestion.* · Strawberry tongue. · Diarrhea, abdominal pain. · Arthritis, carditis, aseptic meningitis.	· Clinical diagnosis (five of six asterisked [*] criteria listed in columns three and four).	· Supportive.
Toxic shock syndrome	· *Staphylococcus aureus*—probably toxin-mediated.	· Diffuse blanching, erythematous macular rash* followed by desquamation* of affected skin, including hands and feet (rash may go unnoticed). · Scattered petechiae, especially in inguinal and antecubital areas.	· Occurs predominantly in menstruating women using tampons. · Fever.* · Hypotension.* · Organ system involvement: gastrointestinal (vomiting, diarrhea); muscular (myalgia, increased creatine phosphokinase); mucous membranes (vaginal, oropharyngeal, or conjunctival hyperemia, strawberry tongue); renal (increased creatinine); hepatic (increased liver function test results); hematologic (decreased platelets); central nervous system abnormalities.	· Clinical diagnosis (all asterisked[*] criteria listed in columns three and four, plus three or more organ systems involved).	· Aggressive supportive care. · Antistaphylococcal antibiotics intravenously.

† Establishing a diagnosis of each of these entities requires exclusion of other diseases that may be associated with scarlatiniform rashes, eg, allergic drug-related eruptions, serum sickness, infectious mononucleosis, rubeola, atypical measles, rubella, roseola, leptospirosis, Rocky Mountain spotted fever.

Scarlet fever and scarlatiniform eruptions

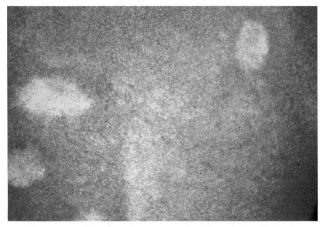

3-1. The rash of scarlet fever is typified by pinhead-sized, discrete, erythematous macules that blanch when pressure is applied.

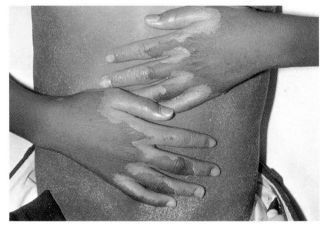

3-2. Generalized desquamation occurs late in the course of scarlet fever.

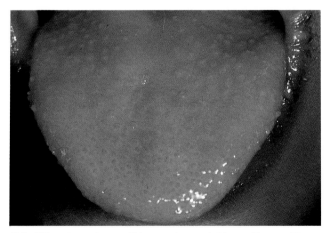

3-3. "Strawberry tongue" is seen in scarlet fever, Kawasaki syndrome, and toxic shock syndrome.

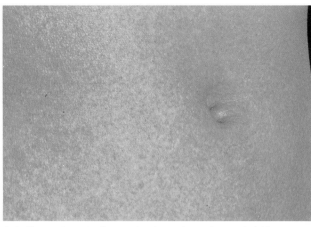

3-4. The early rash of toxic shock syndrome is scarlatiniform.

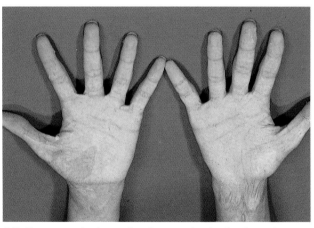

3-5. Desquamation is a salient feature of toxic shock syndrome.

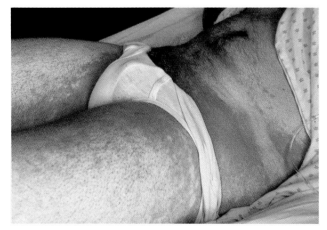

3-6. Although it occurs most often in menstruating women, toxic shock syndrome also occurs in men.

Smooth Papules

Molluscum contagiosum

Skin
- Translucent, pink, or flesh-colored, dome-shaped papules, 2 to 10 mm in diameter (occasionally up to 2 cm), often with central depression (umbilication), are present.
- Some lesions may be excoriated.
- Lesions may occur on any body area except palms and soles and are often asymmetrical.
- Lesions are often grouped.
- Lesions may occur on mucous membranes.
- Eczematous dermatitis may develop in nearby skin.

Pathogenesis
- A benign proliferation of epidermal cells develops in response to infection by a poxvirus.
- Transmission is by direct contact.

Clinical features
- Most infections occur in children.
- Infection is usually asymptomatic but itching may occur.
- There are no systemic signs or symptoms.

Differential diagnosis
- Folliculitis, lichen planus, verrucae, varicella, scabies, excoriated eczema.
- Solitary lesion: keratoacanthoma, pyogenic granuloma, basal cell carcinoma.

Diagnostic tests
- Pressure on lesion may express cheese-like material.
- Center shows black dot if lesions are sprayed with ethyl chloride.
- Giemsa's stain of expressed material demonstrates molluscum bodies.
- Biopsy: histopathology is diagnostic.

Therapy
- Cryotherapy.
- Curettage.
- Keratolytic agents in flexible collodion.
- Sometimes simple expression.
- Usually resolves spontaneously without scarring.

Molluscum contagiosum

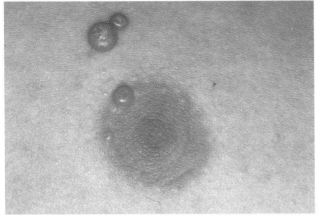

4-1. *The papules of molluscum contagiosum are dome-shaped and often become umbilicated.*

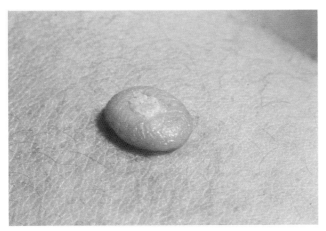

4-2. *In adults, the pubic area is commonly involved.*

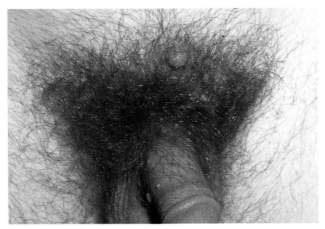

4-3. *Some lesions may grow to several centimeters in diameter.*

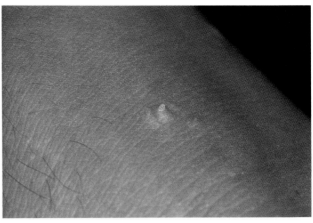

4-4. *Pressure may express a cheese-like white core.*

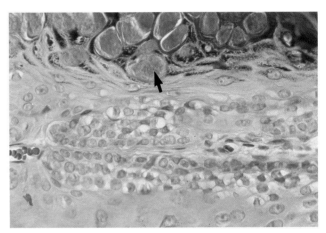

4-5. *Molluscum bodies (arrow) are diagnostic of molluscum contagiosum.*

Smooth Papules

Condyloma latum (secondary syphilis)

Skin
- Hypopigmented, flat-topped, discrete or coalescent papules and plaques occur in intertriginous areas.
- Lesions develop in moist areas, eg, vulva, anus, lip, toe web, or axilla.
- Other cutaneous manifestations of secondary syphilis, such as generalized rash (often papulosquamous), split papules, generalized patchy hair loss, and mucous patches may also be present.

Pathogenesis
- These skin lesions are a manifestation of secondary syphilis.
- Lesions contain *Treponema pallidum*.

Clinical features
- Clinical findings occur one to four months (usually six to eight weeks) after primary chancre appears.
- Mild systemic symptoms such as malaise, headache, anorexia, and sore throat occur.
- Generalized lymphadenopathy (nontender, hard, and large nodes) may also be present.
- Jaundice, nephropathy, iritis, periostitis, myositis, meningismus, and nerve palsies rarely occur.

Differential diagnosis
- Condyloma acuminatum, hemorrhoids.

Diagnostic tests
- Dark-field examination of exudate from lesion.
- Serologic tests for syphilis, including fluorescent treponemal antibody-absorption test for syphilis (FTA-ABS).

Therapy
- Benzathine penicillin.

Condyloma latum (secondary syphilis)

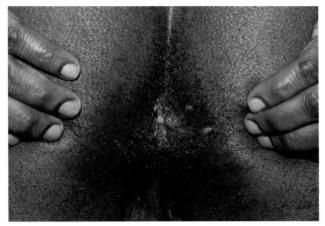

5-1. *In contrast to condyloma acuminatum, the papules of condyloma latum are smoother and softer.*

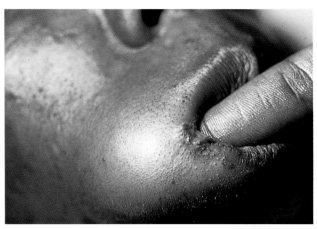

5-4. *Split papules of secondary syphilis are indurated fissures often found at the corners of the mouth or nasolabial folds.*

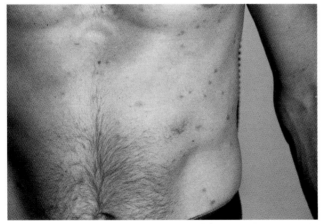

5-2. *The truncal lesions of secondary syphilis may mimic pityriasis rosea or tinea versicolor.*

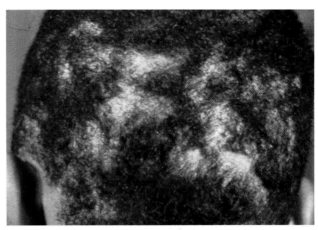

5-5. *"Moth-eaten" alopecia refers to the patchy, diffuse hair loss of secondary syphilis.*

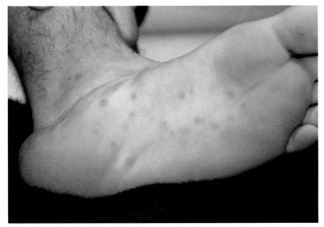

5-3. *Palms and soles are commonly involved in secondary syphilis.*

Verrucous Papules or Plaques

Condyloma acuminatum (venereal warts)

Skin
- Verrucous, vegetative, cauliflower-surfaced, pedunculated, or wide-stalked, keratotic, skin-colored papules are present.
- Coalescence or enlargement can produce disc-like tumors.
- Infection almost always occurs on moist surfaces such as the genitalia, urethra, perianal and rectal tissue, or lips.

Pathogenesis
- Epidermal proliferation is caused by infection with a strain of human papillomavirus.
- It is sometimes transmitted sexually.
- Pregnancy may stimulate growth.

Clinical features
- Infection is limited to the skin and mucous membranes.

Differential diagnosis
- Condyloma latum (of syphilis), squamous cell carcinoma, skin tags, Bowenoid papulosis, seborrheic keratoses.

Diagnostic tests
- Usually a clinical diagnosis.
- Ordinary histopathology suggests the diagnosis.
- Electron microscopy demonstrates characteristic virus in excised tissues.
- Serologic test for syphilis or dark-field examination can help rule out condyloma latum.

Therapy
- 20% podophyllin in tincture of benzoin.
- Electrofulguration.
- Cryosurgery.

Condyloma acuminatum (venereal warts)

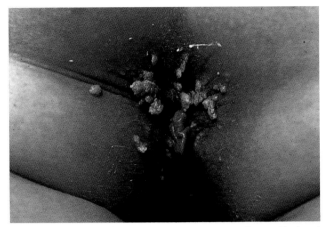

6-1. *Venereal warts typically occur on moist surfaces. Perianal lesions are often associated with anal intercourse.*

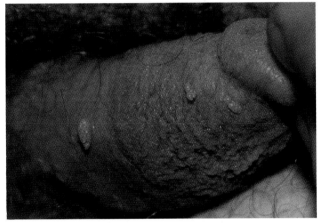

6-2. *Accuminate papules often appear on the penis.*

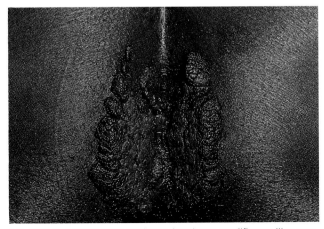

6-3. *Perianal warts may coalesce into large cauliflower-like masses and involve the anal canal.*

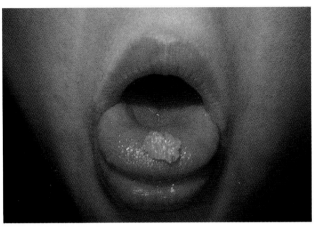

6-4. *Warts may develop on the tongue, lips, or other mucous membranes.*

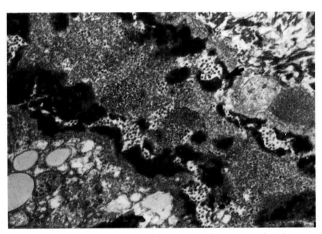

6-5. *The virus that causes condyloma acuminatum can be demonstrated by electronmicroscopy (arrow).*

Verrucous Papules or Plaques

Verrucae

Skin

Verruca vulgaris (common wart)

- Hard, elevated, keratotic papules with a rough, velvet-textured, or vegetated surface develop.
- Papules are usually 2 to 10 mm in diameter but may be much larger.
- Warts tend to occur on the hands but may affect any body site.
- One, two, or many lesions may be present.

Verruca plana (flat wart)

- Flat-topped, nonscaling, skin-colored papules 2 to 4 mm in diameter develop.
- Flat warts usually occur on hands, neck, or face.
- Lesions are almost always multiple and grouped.

Verruca plantaris (plantar wart)

- Flat to slightly elevated, well-defined, slightly yellow keratotic papules develop, usually on soles of feet.
- Papules are occasionally studded with black dots.
- Multiple lesions may become confluent (mosaic wart).

Verruca filiformis (filiform wart)

- A horn-like, thin-stalked, keratotic papilloma develops, usually on face or neck.

Condyloma acuminatum (discussed in preceding section).

Pathogenesis

- Epidermal proliferation is caused by infection with human papillomavirus of various strains.
- Different strains cause different types of warts.
- Transmission is by direct contact or autoinoculation.

Clinical features

- Features are limited to the skin and mucous membranes.

Differential diagnosis

- *Verruca vulgaris:* seborrheic keratosis, actinic keratosis.
- *Verruca plana:* lichen planus, lichen nitidus, molluscum contagiosum.
- *Verruca plantaris:* corns, calluses, squamous cell carcinoma, calcaneal petechiae.
- *Verruca filiformis:* cutaneous horns, seborrheic keratosis.

Diagnostic tests

- Usually a clinical diagnosis.
- Ordinary histopathology is diagnostic or often suggestive of verrucae.
- Electron microscopy demonstrates characteristic virus in excised lesions.

Therapy

- Cryosurgery.
- Keratolytic ointments, plasters, solutions.
- Curettage.
- Electrodesiccation.
- Destructive acids.

Verrucae

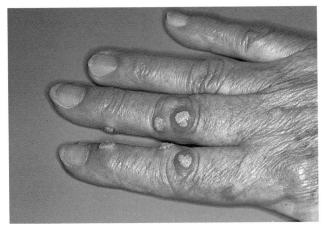

7-1. The common wart is a hard papule with a rough surface. These "kissing warts" may have spread by direct contact.

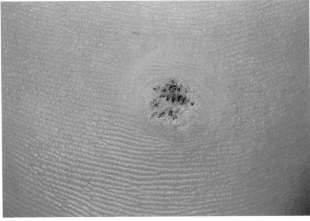

7-4. When pared, plantar warts are usually studded with small black dots or bleeding points.

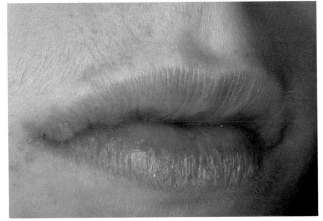

7-2. Flat warts are usually numerous and grouped on the neck, face, or hands.

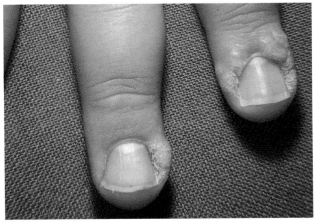

7-5. Periungual warts morphologically resemble common warts but occur around the nails.

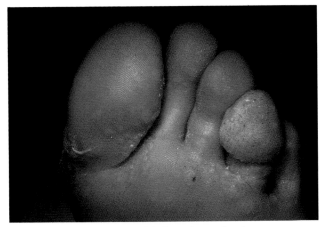

7-3. Plantar warts are yellowish, hyperkeratotic plaques.

Verrucous Papules or Plaques

Cutaneous tuberculosis

Disease	Skin	Pathogenesis	Clinical features	Differential diagnosis
Primary inoculation tuberculosis	· Papule becomes a shallow, painless, undermined, red-blue ulcer with irregular or hemorrhagic base, often studded with tiny pustules. · Later, the ulcer becomes nodular. · The ulcer usually occurs on the hand.	· Infection results from primary inoculation of *Mycobacterium tuberculosis;* inoculation through wounds is possible.	· There are usually no systemic symptoms. · Regional adenopathy. · Rarely may disseminate. · Erythema nodosum (10% of cases).	· Primary syphilis, tularemia, sporotrichosis, atypical mycobacterial infection, orf, milker's nodule, anthrax, carcinoma, deep fungus infection.
Tuberculosis verrucosa cutis	· A papule becomes a hyperkeratotic verrucous papule or plaque, which may fissure. · The lesion usually occurs on the hand.	· Infection results from inoculation of *M tuberculosis* in persons previously sensitized; inoculation through wounds is possible.	· Usually no adenopathy occurs.	· Warts, seborrheic keratosis, blastomycosis, bromoderma, chromomycosis, atypical AFB,* lichen planus.
Lupus vulgaris	· Brown-to-red, soft, smooth, rounded papules, solitary or multiple, are present, usually on the head or neck. · Occasionally they are serpiginous, psoriasiform, tumorous, or ulcerative. · Prominent scars may result.	· Infection may result from dissemination—usually from cervical adenitis, inoculation reexposure, or primary tuberculosis in nodes, lung, or elsewhere. · Satellite lesions coalesce.	· Infection may destroy cartilage and may induce carcinoma.	· Rosacea, sarcoid, leprosy, blastomycosis, bromoderma, chromomycosis, atypical AFB,* neoplasm, gumma.

*Acid-fast bacteria

Diagnostic tests	Purified protein derivative (PPD) skin test	Therapy
Biopsy with stain for AFB.* Smear. Culture.	• Negative or positive.	• Antituberculous chemotherapy.

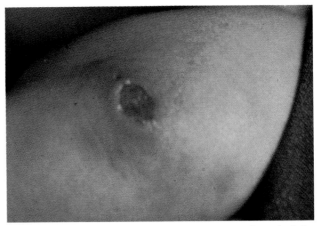

8-1. *The border of the ulcer of primary inoculation tuberculosis is commonly undermined.*

Biopsy for culture.	• Positive.	• Excision. • Antituberculous chemotherapy.

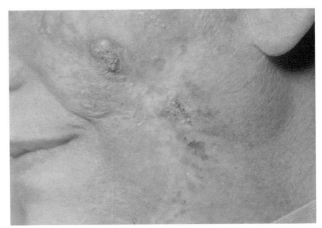

8-2. *These red papules of lupus vulgaris have an apple-jelly color when blanched with a glass slide.*

Upon pressure of papule with glass slide, papule turns to color of apple jelly. Culture.	• Positive.	• Excision. • Antituberculous chemotherapy.

8-3. *Scarring is a prominent feature of late lupus vulgaris, and squamous cell carcinoma may develop, as in this patient.*

Verrucous Papules or Palaques

Cutaneous tuberculosis

Disease	Skin	Pathogenesis	Clinical features	Differential diagnosis
Scrofuloderma	· Firm subcutaneous nodules become ulcers and sinuses with undermined, purple borders and granulating bases.	· Initial infection, often of cervical nodes, may be a result of drinking unpasteurized milk or a result of direct spread to skin from underlying tuberculosis of node, bone, joint, or other tissue; it may occasionally be spread by hematogenous dissemination.	· Usually children are affected.	· Hidradenitis suppurativa, gumma, sporotrichosis, facticial ulcer.
Miliary tuberculosis	· Pinhead-sized macules or papules develop and are pink, skin-colored, or purpuric and cover the entire body, especially the trunk.	· Hematogenous, widespread dissemination from a primary or reactivated focus of tuberculosis.	· Usually infants or severely debilitated persons are affected.	· Milia, scarlatiniform rashes, miliaria.

*Acid-fast bacteria.

gnostic ts	Purified protein derivative (PPD) skin test	Therapy
xamine underlying ne, joint, or des.	· Positive.	· Antituberculous chemotherapy.
ulture.		
iopsy with stain for FB.*		

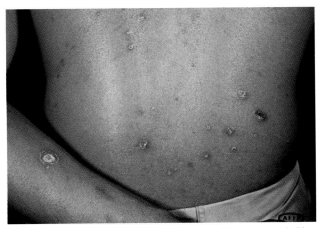

8-4. *Papulonecrotic tuberculid is a disseminated, ulcerated skin eruption associated with tuberculosis, but it does not usually contain mycobacterial organisms.*

iopsy with stain for FB.*	· May be negative.	· Antituberculous chemotherapy.
ulture.		

8-5. *Biopsy specimens may show acid-fast bacilli.*

Verrucous Papules or Plaques

Blastomycosis

Skin
- Papulopustular lesions gradually enlarge and become raised, verrucous, and crusted.
- Lesions characteristically advance peripherally, with abruptly slanted borders and central healing.
- Lesions start on exposed areas (face, hands, lower legs).
- Multiple lesions develop in the majority of cases.

Pathogenesis
- The disease is caused by *Blastomyces dermatitidis*, a dimorphic fungus.
- The portal of entry is the respiratory tract; infection most commonly spreads to the skin (80% of cases), bones, and genitourinary tract (prostate, testes, and epididymis).

Clinical features
- Males are affected more often than are females; persons 30 to 50 years old are affected most often.
- Endemic areas are the Middle Atlantic and Southeastern United States, Mississippi Valley, and upper Midwest.
- The onset is insidious with malaise, fever, productive cough, and development of chronic pneumonia (chest x-ray results are not distinctive).
- Skin lesions (in 25% to 40% of cases at outset), osteomyelitis, orchitis, and epididymitis may also be present.
- The disease may be limited to one organ (especially the lung or skin).

Differential diagnosis
- Often mistaken for squamous cell carcinoma; can be confused with sporotrichosis, tuberculosis, syphilis, iododerma, bromoderma, or pulmonary lesions of tuberculosis, histoplasmosis, coccidioidomycosis, nocardiosis, or carcinoma.

Diagnostic tests
- Biopsy periphery of skin lesion with special stains (eg, Gomori's methenamine silver) and culture (Sabouraud's agar).
- Trained microscopist can recognize typical budding yeasts in biopsy specimen.
- Potassium-hydroxide-treated preparations of exudates (sputum, pus, prostatic massage fluid) for identification of yeast forms (presumptive diagnosis).
- Definitive diagnosis by culture (may take four to eight weeks for isolation and final identification).

Therapy
- Amphotericin B intravenously.
- Occasionally a patient may not need treatment if clinical improvement has already occurred.

Blastomycosis

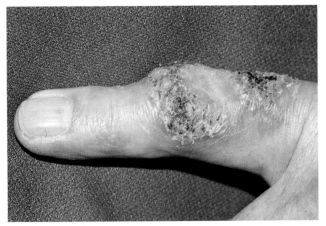

9-1. The characteristic lesion is an inflamed nodular plaque with a wart-like surface and central healing.

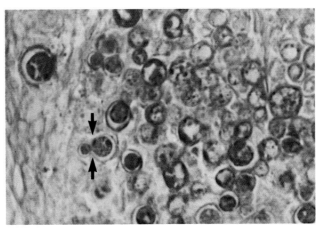

9-4. The yeast of blastomycosis typically has a broad-based bud.

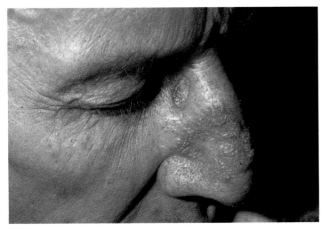

9-2. Lesions most typically begin on exposed body surfaces.

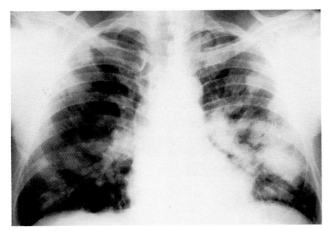

9-3. The primary site of infection is usually the lungs.

Verrucous Papules or Plaques

Coccidioidomycosis

Skin
- Morphology is variable: papules, pustules, plaques, nodules, ulcers, or abscesses may be present.
- Most commonly, irregularly surfaced or verrucous plaques or nodules, often ulcerated, develop.
- Erythema nodosum (discussed in section titled Erythematous Patches or Nodules) or erythema multiforme (discussed in section titled Serpiginous or Annular Plaques) may be present.

Pathogenesis
- Infection is caused by hematogenous dissemination of the fungus *Coccidioides immitis* from a primary pulmonary site to the skin; direct inoculation of skin (eg, laboratory accident) rarely occurs.
- Granulomatous tissue reaction develops.

Clinical features
- Persons who reside in or travel to an endemic area, eg, Southwestern United States or Northern Mexico, are at risk of infection.
- Patient may have evidence of coccidioidomycosis elsewhere, eg, pulmonary, meningeal, or musculoskeletal disease.

Differential diagnosis
- Cutaneous tuberculosis, syphilis, blastomycosis, actinomycosis, staphylococcal pyoderma, cryptococcosis.

Diagnostic tests
- Potassium hydroxide (KOH) preparation of soft-tissue aspirates, sputum, or pus (spherules with endospores are characteristic) or Gomori's methenamine silver stain of skin biopsy.
- Culture (Sabouraud's medium).
- Elevated complement-fixation antibody titers suggest disseminated disease.
- Skin tests not helpful for diagnosis.

Therapy
- Disseminated disease: systemic amphotericin B.
- Single lesions of direct inoculation: consider excision.

Coccidioidomycosis

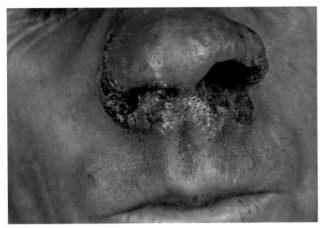

10-1. *One of the most typical cutaneous manifestations of cocci-dioidomycosis is a vegetative, verrucous plaque.*

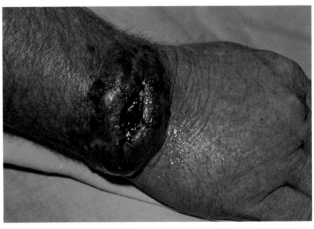

10-4. *Granulomatous pyodermas may resemble coccidioidomy-cosis.*

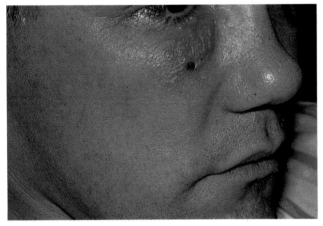

10-2. *Here, coccidioidomycosis appears as an irregularly sur-faced plaque.*

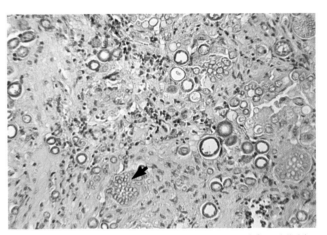

10-5. *Characteristic spherules with endospores of Coccidioides immitis are seen in this tissue-biopsy specimen.*

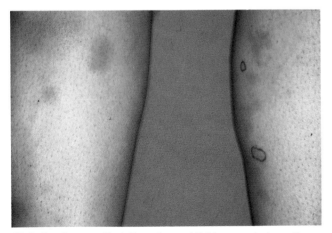

10-3. *Another manifestation of coccidioidomycosis is erythema nodosum.*

Verrucous Papules or Plaques

Chromomycosis

Skin

- Verrucous papule or vegetating ulcer, usually on exposed skin, especially feet and legs, develops into verrucous nodules or tumors.
- Verrucous, hyperkeratotic papules may become verrucous ulcers and plaques.
- Satellite papules and ulcers coalesce to huge plaques with a prominent verrucous surface.
- Lesions are slowly progressive and may last for years, but they may resolve centrally to heal with scarring.

Pathogenesis

- Infection of skin and subcutaneous tissue is caused by fungi of the *Phialophora, Cladosporium,* or *Fonsecaea* species.
- A penetrating injury often causes inoculation of the pathogenic organism.

Clinical features

- Most patients are adult agricultural workers living in rural, tropical areas.
- Infection is usually limited to the skin.
- Brain abscesses with or without cutaneous lesions may rarely occur.

Differential diagnosis

- Iododerma, bromoderma, mycosis fungoides, viral verrucae, blastomycosis, tuberculosis verrucosa cutis, syphilis, yaws, leishmaniasis, psoriasis, sporotrichosis.

Diagnostic tests

- Potassium hydroxide (KOH) examination or biopsy for brown thick-walled organisms, often in clusters.
- Culture.

Therapy

- Surgical removal of early lesions.
- Systemic 5-fluorocytosine.
- Amphotericin B (?)
- Thiabendazole (?)

Chromomycosis

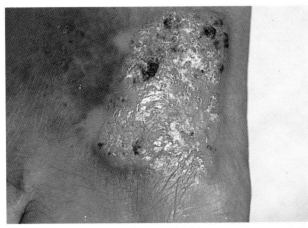

11-1. *Chromomycosis is characterized by verrucous, vegetative, ulcerated tumors.*

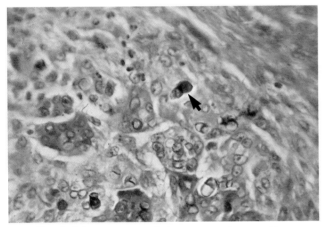

11-2. *The dark-brown spores of chromomycosis resemble copper pennies.*

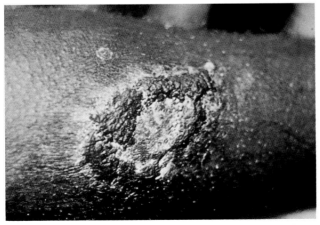

11-3. *Cutaneous leishmaniasis can resemble chromomycosis.*

Wheals

Urticaria

Skin
- Transient pink papules and plaques, without overlying epidermal change, develop.
- Individual wheals appear quickly and disappear within 24 hours without scar or pigment change.
- Wheals usually itch.
- The eruption is usually generalized, affecting all areas of the skin.

Pathogenesis
- Urticaria is a reaction pattern often associated with allergy, but it can also be due to physical, hereditary, chemical, or emotional causes.
- Infection is a common cause; associated infections include respiratory viruses, hepatitis, infectious mononucleosis, *Mycoplasma pneumoniae* infections, urinary tract infections, abscessed teeth, sinusitis, and parasitic infection of the bowel.

Clinical features
- Findings are dependent on the site of infection and the nature of the infecting organism.

Differential diagnosis
- Physical and hereditary urticaria, urticaria from noninfectious causes (such as drugs), bites, dermatitis herpetiformis, pruritic urticarial papules and plaques of pregnancy, acute allergic contact dermatitis, mastocytosis.
- Urticarial vasculitis mimics urticaria and may be accompanied by joint pain and nephritis.

Diagnostic tests
- Good history and physical examination with appropriate laboratory tests.
- Thorough survey for occult infection, ordinarily indicated only if urticaria persists three or more months.
- Dependent on suspected etiologic agent.

Therapy
- Treat or remove cause.
- Antihistamines.
- Sympathomimetics.
- Rarely, systemic corticosteroids.

Urticaria

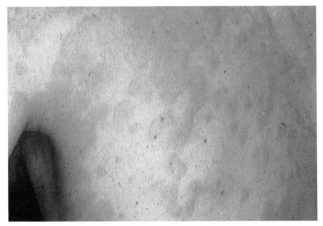

12-1. *Urticarial wheals are pruritic, erythematous, edematous papules without scales.*

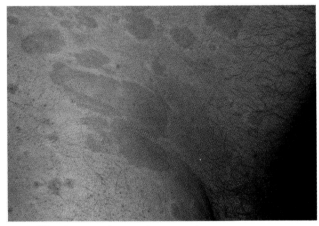

12-2. *Wheals may enlarge to become plaques.*

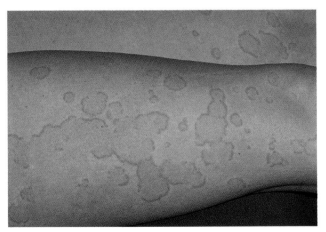

12-3. *Plaques may clear centrally and form annular lesions resembling erythema multiforme.*

Wheals

Scabies

Skin
- Symmetrical, severely pruritic, erythematous papules develop, which often quickly become excoriated.
- Flexor wrists, finger webs, axillary folds, glans penis, and nipples are especially predisposed areas.
- The head is spared, except in children.
- Burrows are short, wavy, elongated papules.
- Secondary eczematous dermatitis is fairly common.
- Brown-to-red pruritic nodules sometimes develop on covered areas.

Pathogenesis
- Infection is caused by the mite *Sarcoptes scabiei* var *hominis*.
- Eruption and itch are caused by an immune reaction to mites, mite eggs, or mite feces.
- Transmission is by body-to-body contact.

Clinical features
- Findings are limited to the skin.

Differential diagnosis
- Excoriated eczema, dermatitis herpetiformis, papular urticaria, neurotic excoriations, arthropod bites, papular dermatitis of infancy.

Diagnostic tests
- Scrape burrow with scalpel blade covered with mineral oil, smear on slide, and examine microscopically for mites, mite eggs, or mite feces.

Therapy
- Gamma benzene hexachloride cream or lotion.
- Crotamiton lotion.
- 5% to 10% precipitated sulfur in petrolatum.
- Household and sexual contacts usually should be treated.

Scabies

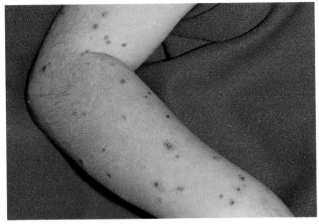

13-1. *The most prominent feature of scabies is a widespread eruption of pruritic, excoriated papules.*

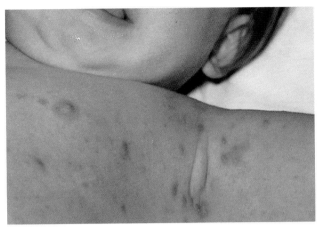

13-4. *Sometimes nodules develop.*

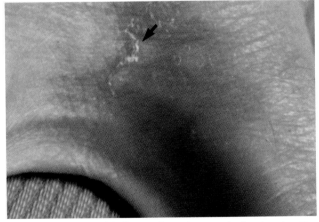

13-2. *The most helpful diagnostic cutaneous lesion is a burrow (arrow).*

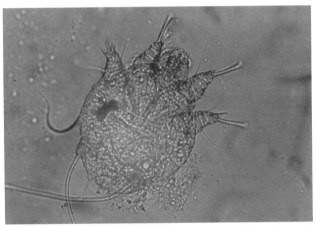

13-5. *Sarcoptes scabiei can frequently be extracted from the end of a burrow.*

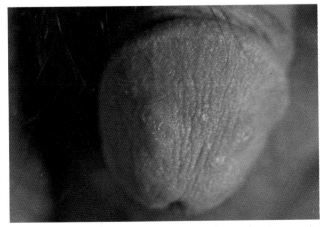

13-3. *Lesions commonly occur on flexor surfaces, the glans penis, and areolae.*

Cercarial dermatitis (swimmer's itch)

Skin
- The patient begins to itch while in the water or shortly thereafter.
- Transient pink macules or papules appear within one hour, then later subside.
- Four to 48 hours later, diffuse pruritic erythematous papules appear and become ulcerated from excoriation.
- Infection occurs only on skin exposed to the water, with relative sparing of the bathing suit area.
- Infection resolves after three to 14 days.

Pathogenesis
- Penetration of the skin by cercariae (immature larvae) of avian or mammalian schistosomes (blood flukes) produces the papules.
- Snails discharge *Trichobilharzia stagnicolae* or other species that float in water and adhere, with ventral suckers, to the skin.
- Eruption usually occurs after the patient has been swimming or wading in fresh water during spring or summer.
- Cercariae penetrate the skin and may produce immediate erythema.
- Diffuse pruritic papules that appear four to 48 hours later are a manifestation of a delayed hypersensitivity reaction at the site of penetration.
- Man is an incidental host.

Clinical features
- Findings are limited to the skin.

Differential diagnosis
- Scabies, arthropod bites, sea bather's eruption.

Diagnostic tests
- Clinical diagnosis.

Therapy
- Dry skin briskly with a rough towel if contact is suspected.
- Symptomatic.
- Avoid infested water.

Cercarial dermatitis (swimmer's itch)

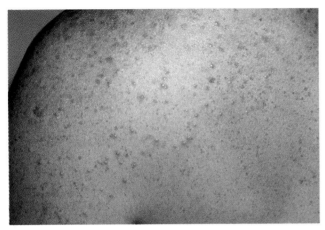

14-1. *Diffuse pruritic papules of swimmer's itch develop within one to two days after the person has been swimming in infested water.*

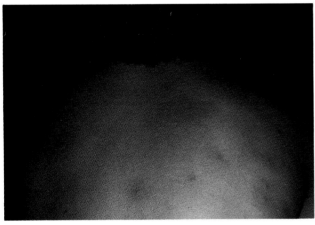

14-2. *The erythematous flare in this patient is pronounced.*

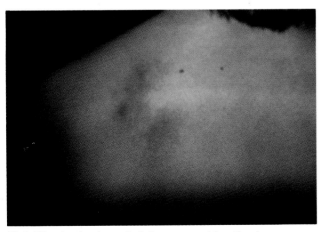

14-3. *Wheals of swimmer's itch can resemble urticaria.*

Serpiginous or Annular Plaques

Erythema multiforme

Skin

- Symmetrical urticarial papules suddenly appear over any body area, especially the extremities.
- Palms and soles are commonly affected.
- Papules enlarge to form annular plaques.
- New papules may develop in the center of annular plaques to create "target" (iris) lesions.
- Mucous membrane involvement heralds Stevens-Johnson syndrome in which skin lesions may become bullous.

Pathogenesis

- Hypersensitivity reaction develops to infection, drugs, chemicals, or other factors.
- Associated infections include herpes simplex, herpes zoster, orf, milker's nodules, coxsackie B5, echoviruses, influenza type A, poliomyelitis, adenovirus, mumps, lymphogranuloma venereum, *Streptococcus, Staphylococcus, Salmonella, Pseudomonas,* histoplasmosis, coccidioidomycosis, mycobacteria, syphilis, *Trichomonas,* and vaccinia.

Clinical features

- Usually only the skin is affected.
- Stevens-Johnson syndrome is the triad of (1) erythema multiforme, (2) mucous membrane involvement (conjunctivitis, stomatitis, urethritis, bronchitis), and (3) constitutional symptoms, such as fever, headache, and malaise. Rarely, glomerulonephritis, myocarditis, pericarditis, pneumonia, intestinal bleeding, encephalitis, arthritis, and death may occur.

Differential diagnosis

- Atypical measles, annular urticaria, Rocky Mountain spotted fever, toxic epidermal necrolysis, erythema marginatum (a more serpiginous eruption associated with rheumatic fever).

Diagnostic tests

- Biopsy: histopathology relatively specific for erythema multiforme.
- Search for infection.

Therapy

- Treat or remove cause.
- Systemic corticosteroids.
- Antihistamines.
- Wet compresses.

Erythema multiforme

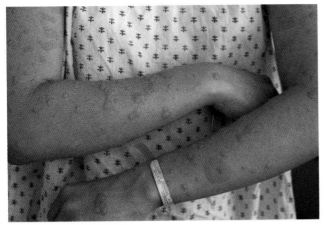

15-1. *Initially, erythema multiforme resembles urticaria.*

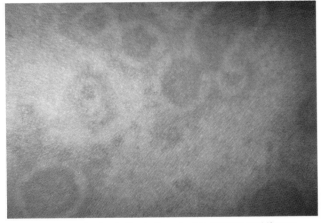

15-2. *The target lesion is the hallmark of erythema multiforme.*

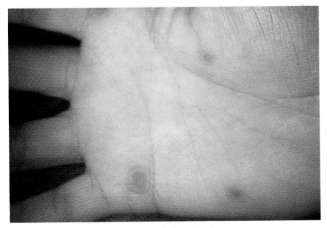

15-3. *Palms and soles are usually involved.*

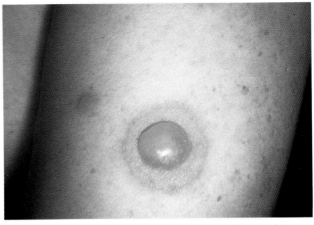

15-4. *Tense bullae may develop, especially in Stevens-Johnson syndrome.*

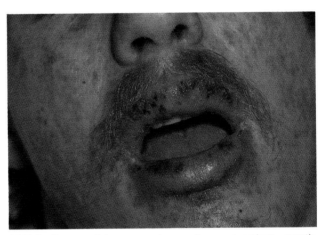

15-5. *In Stevens-Johnson syndrome, the conjunctivae, mouth, and tracheobronchial tree may be affected.*

Serpiginous or Annular Plaques

Erythema chronicum migrans (Lyme disease)

Skin
- A small indurated red macule progresses to form a papule, then an annular plaque.
- A red ring enlarges up to 50 cm in diameter; a large bright-red to blue-red ring with paler interior is characteristic of erythema chronicum migrans.
- A punctum from the bite may be present at the center of the ring.
- Multiple secondary lesions may develop.
- Lesions commonly occur on the thigh or buttock or near the axilla.
- The lesions may last days to months.

Pathogenesis
- A tick (Ixodes dammini) apparently acts as a vector to transmit infection by an as yet unidentified agent.
- Genetic predisposition to some complications is probable.
- Immune complexes may be important.

Clinical features
- Onset occurs May through August in endemic areas (primarily New England), but sporadic cases can occur elsewhere.
- Fever, headache, malaise, and stiff neck may be present.
- Joint involvement may develop and be recurrent (beginning within several days or up to years after the tick bite).
- Neurologic and cardiac disorders are variable and develop a few weeks after the bite; they are not recurrent.

Differential diagnosis
- Skin lesions: tinea corporis, granuloma annulare, erythema annulare centrifugum, tick bite hypersensitivity reaction.
- Arthritis can mimic other forms of arthritis, eg, rheumatoid arthritis.

Diagnostic test
- Clinical diagnosis.
- Cryoglobulinemia may predict the development of arthritis.

Therapy
- Penicillin or tetracycline.

Erythema chronicum migrans (Lyme disease)

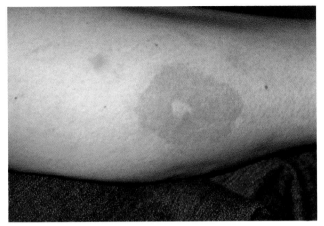

16-1. *Erythema chronicum migrans appears as an enlarging bright-red annular plaque.*

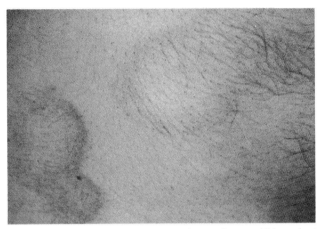

16-4. *Not every annular skin lesion is Lyme disease. This patient has granuloma annulare.*

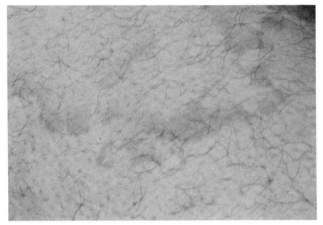

16-2. *Later, lesions may become serpiginous.*

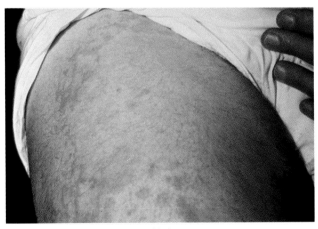

16-3. *Lesions may become multiple.*

Serpiginous or Annular Plaques

Cutaneous larva migrans (creeping eruption)

Skin
- One or more raised, erythematous, tubular, serpiginous lesions 2 to 3 mm wide are characteristic.
- Lesions contain serous fluid, and crust may form on the surface.
- Lesions extend 1 to 2 cm per day.
- A tingling skin sensation occurs at the time of larva penetration.
- Any site of the body can be involved, but usually the lesions occur on the feet or buttocks.
- The lesion is intensely pruritic.

Pathogenesis
- Larva of nematodes (usually nonhuman pathogens, eg, *Ancylostoma braziliense*–dog and cat hookworm) penetrate the skin and migrate underneath the epidermis.
- Humans are abnormal hosts, so the disease is confined to the skin (in contrast to visceral larva migrans, which is caused by other hookworm species).

Clinical features
- The disease usually occurs in persons in the southern United States.
- All ages are affected.
- Children, farmers, gardeners, and swimmers are at greater risk of exposure.

Differential diagnosis
- Granuloma annulare, poison ivy.

Diagnostic tests
- Usually a clinical diagnosis.
- Recovery of worm by skin biopsy is difficult.

Therapy
- Topical or systemic thiabendazole.

Cutaneous larva migrans (creeping eruption)

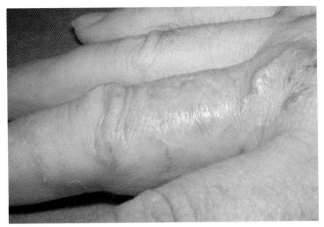

17-1. *Creeping eruption is characterized by an advancing linear or serpiginous plaque.*

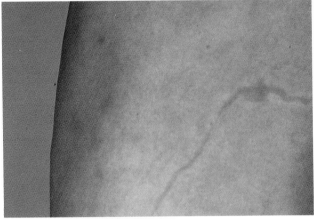

17-2. *This is a striking example of cutaneous larva migrans.*

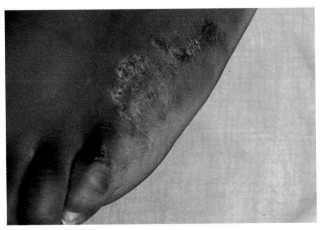

17-3. *The foot is a common location.*

Erythematous Patches or Nodules

Erythema infectiosum (fifth disease)

Skin

- Pink macules and papules on the cheeks coalesce and progress to confluent marked erythema resembling a slapped cheek—hot but not tender.
- Central clearing creates a net-like (reticulated) pattern.
- Two to four days later, pink macules and papules occur over the trunk and extremities, especially the shoulders, and these coalesce to form a net-like pattern.
- Lesions are evanescent and recurrent but fade after six to ten days.

Pathogenesis

- The disease has a presumed viral cause.
- It occurs in epidemics, especially in winter or spring.

Clinical features

- The disease usually affects children.
- Prodrome is either absent or mild (headache, malaise, nausea, and muscle aching).
- Early: mild leukocytosis with relative lymphocytopenia occurs.
- Later: eosinophilia and sometimes lymphocytosis occur.
- Encephalitis, pneumonitis, and hemolytic anemia rarely occur.

Differential diagnosis

- Flushing, chapping, irritant dermatitis, cellulitis, and especially erysipelas, scarlet fever, rubeola, rubella, sunburn, lupus erythematosus, or drug-related eruption.

Diagnostic tests

- Clinical diagnosis.
- No specific tests need to be performed.

Therapy

- Symptomatic.

Erythema infectiosum (fifth disease)

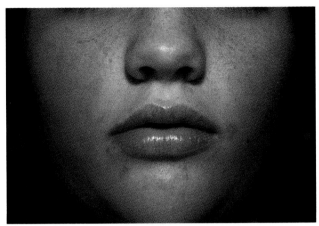

18-1. *The rosy, "slapped cheek" appearance of early fifth disease is often overlooked.*

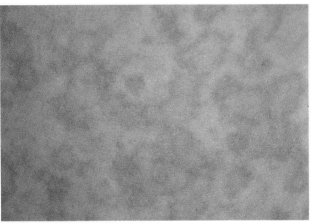

18-4. *Later, the arms and trunk may become affected.*

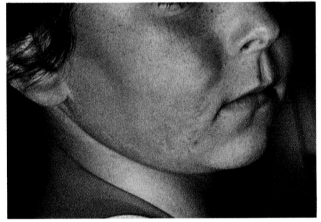

18-2. *In other patients, the cheeks may become bright red.*

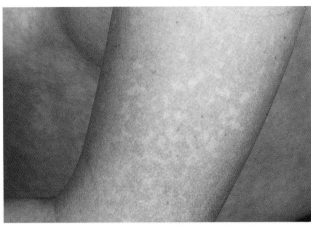

18-5. *The erythema, especially on the shoulders, has a net-like appearance.*

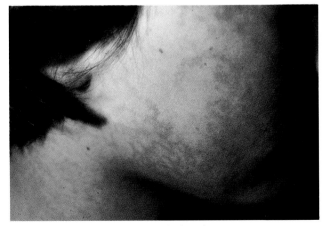

18-3. *Central clearing gives a reticulated pattern.*

Erythematous Patches or Nodules

Streptococcal cellulitis

Skin
- A tender, warm, erythematous, edematous unilateral patch or plaque develops.
- It rapidly enlarges.
- It may be accompanied by lymphangitis (red, tender, linear streaks directed toward enlarged, tender lymph nodes).
- Erysipelas (a form of streptococcal cellulitis), characterized by raised, demarcated, bright-red areas (usually on the face but can occur anywhere), may develop, and it may be pruritic or painful.

Pathogenesis
- Group A *Streptococcus* (rarely other streptococcal groups) is the most common cause of cellulitis.
- Bacteria may enter the skin at a wound or burn site, but often the entry site is inapparent.
- Erysipelas is a dermal and subcutaneous infection.

Clinical features
- Infection may occur at any age.
- Usually patients experience an abrupt onset of fever, chills, headache, and malaise.

Differential diagnosis
- Cellulitis from other pyogenic bacteria (especially *Staphylococcus aureus,* occasionally *Hemophilus influenzae)*.
- Synergistic cellulitis (see next section).
- Erysipeloid (a cellulitis that occurs most often in handlers of saltwater fish or meats, caused by *Erysipelothrix rhusiopathiae)*.
- Cellulitis due to *Aeromonas hydrophila* (occurs by laceration inoculation in fresh water).
- Cellulitis in immunosuppressed host may be due to a variety of opportunistic bacteria and fungi, eg, gram-negative bacilli, *Cryptococcus neoformans.*
- Lupus erythematosus, early herpes zoster, allergic contact dermatitis, giant urticaria, physical injury, arthropod bite.

Diagnostic tests
- Usually a clinical diagnosis.
- Gram stain and culture of skin tissue.
- Blood cultures.

Therapy
- Parenteral penicillin (penicillinase-resistant penicillin or a cephalosporin may be indicated if there is doubt about presence of *S aureus)*.

Streptococcal cellulitis

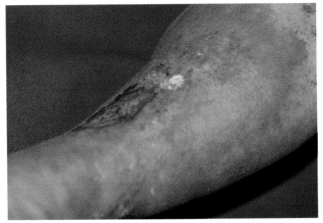

19-1. *In this patient, cellulitis developed in an area of stasis dermatitis and stasis ulcer.*

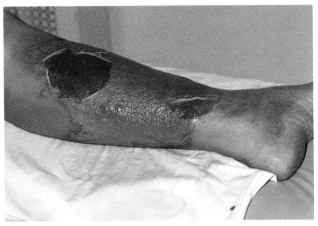

19-4. *Streptococcal cellulitis occasionally becomes bullous.*

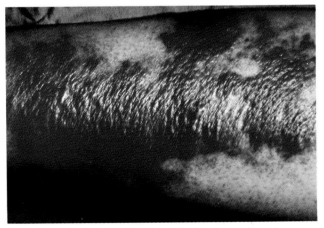

19-2. *Erysipelas, caused by group A streptococci, is characterized by raised, bright-red plaques with sharply defined borders.*

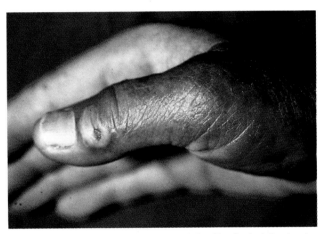

19-5. *Erysipeloid, a cellulitis caused by Erysipelothrix rhusiopathiae, usually occurs on the hands.*

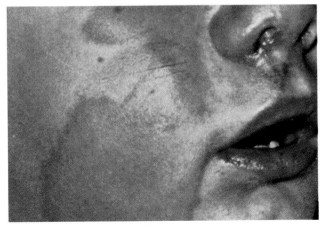

19-3. *Erysipelas commonly affects the face.*

Erythematous Patches or Nodules

Necrotizing (gangrenous) cellulitis

Disease	Skin	Other tissues involved	Organisms	Predisposing conditions	Pain
Synergistic necrotizing cellulitis	• Appearance: Scattered areas of necrosis. • Common location: Perineum, legs. • Gas: Moderate.	• Deeper compartments, including muscle.	• Anaerobes and aerobes.	• Diabetes. • Perirectal infection.	• Severe.
Necrotizing fasciitis	• Appearance: Erythematous cellulitis. • Common location: Wounds. • Gas: Moderate.	• Fascia.	• Group A streptococci, *S aureus*, anaerobes.	• Diabetes. • Abdominal surgery.	• Marked.
Progressive bacterial synergistic gangrene	• Appearance: Central ulcer, surrounding purple hue, outer erythema. • Common location: Wounds. • Gas: Minimal.	• Subcutaneous tissues.	• Microaerophilic streptococci and *S aureus* (or enteric gram-negative bacilli).	• Laparotomy with steel sutures.	• Marked.
Nonclostridial anaerobic cellulitis	• Appearance: Minimal discoloration. • Common location: Wounds. • Gas: Marked.	• Subcutaneous tissues.	• Anaerobes or coliforms or both.	• Diabetes.	• Moderate.

ystemic xicity	Course	Therapy
Severe.	• Rapid.	• Emergency surgery. • Antibiotics.
Marked.	• Rapid.	• Emergency surgery. • Antibiotics.
Minimal.	• Slowly progressive.	• Surgery. • Antibiotics.
Moderate.	• Variable.	• Surgery. • Antibiotics.

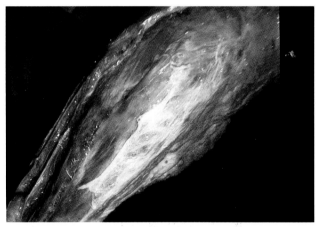

20-1. *Synergistic necrotizing cellulitis commonly involves the perineum and is rapidly progressive.*

20-2. *Necrotizing fasciitis developed in this patient after trauma, necessitating emergency surgery.*

Erythematous Patches or Nodules

Necrotizing (gangrenous) cellulitis

Disease	Skin	Other tissues involved	Organisms	Predisposing conditions	Pain
Clostridial cellulitis	· Appearance: Minimal discoloration. · Common location: Wounds. · Gas: Marked.	· Subcutaneous tissues.	· Clostridial species.	· Local trauma or surgery.	· Moderate.
Clostridial myonecrosis (gas gangrene)	· Appearance: Yellow-bronze, dark bullae. · Common location: Wounds. · Gas: Moderate.	· Muscle.	· Clostridial species.	· Local trauma or surgery.	· Severe.

ystemic xicity	Course	Therapy
Minimal.	• Variable.	• Emergency surgery.
		• Antibiotics.
Severe.	• Rapid.	• Emergency surgery.
		• Antibiotics.
		• Hyperbaric oxygen.

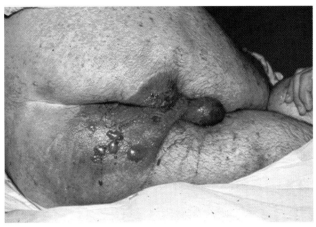

20-3. *Prominent features of clostridial myonecrosis are extensive ecchymoses and necrosis with multiple bullae.*

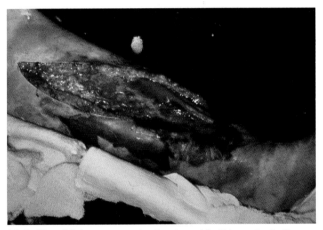

20-4. *Clostridial myonecrosis developed in this patient after an open fracture.*

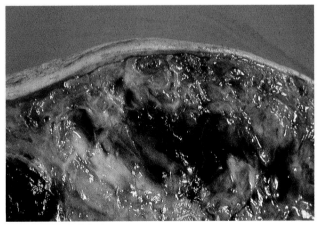

20-5. *Gas gangrene of the abdominal wall followed an elective colectomy for carcinoma of the colon in this patient.*

Erythematous Patches or Nodules

Actinomycosis

Skin

- Infection is characterized by progressive, woody-hard swelling at angle of jaw ("lumpy jaw"), parotid region, or neck. Sinus tracts develop and drain purulent material (cervicofacial actinomycosis); the infection may be painful and fluctuant.
- Thoracic, abdominal, and pelvic actinomycosis may be associated with local indurated swelling of the skin, with sinus tracts.
- A hallmark is the presence of sulfur granules (masses of organisms appearing as yellow or white concretions, up to 2 mm in diameter) in purulent material draining from a sinus tract.

Pathogenesis

- *Actinomyces israelii* (rarely other species), a gram-positive filamentous, anaerobic bacterium, may enter tissue damaged by trauma, surgery, or infection.
- Areas of suppuration have central loculations that contain organisms.
- Sinus tracts extend externally to skin or internally to tongue, larynx, orbit, bone, or other tissues.

Clinical features

- Persons of all ages are affected; males are affected more often than are females.
- Often there is a recent history of dental infection or dental work; cervicofacial, thoracic (aspiration), abdominal, or pelvic infection; or abdominal or pelvic surgery.
- Sometimes fever, weight loss, and fatigue occur.

Differential diagnosis

- Sinus tracts or sulfur granules or both: tuberculosis or staphylococcal, nocardial, and fungal infections.
- Masses without sinus tracts: furuncle, carbuncle, lymphoma, cyst.

Diagnostic tests

- Anaerobic culture of exudate, excised tissue, or sulfur granules.
- Gram stain of exudate and tissue shows gram-positive, filamentous, branching organisms; unlike *Nocardia, Actinomyces* is anaerobic and is not acid fast.
- Hematoxylin and eosin (H and E) stain of excised tissue may show typical ray fungus.

Therapy

- Prolonged course of penicillin or tetracycline.
- Incision and drainage of abscesses.

Actinomycosis

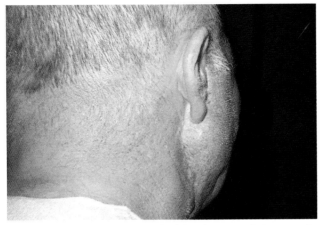

21-1. *The lumpy jaw of cervicofacial actinomycosis is a woody-hard irregular mass near the angle of the mandible.*

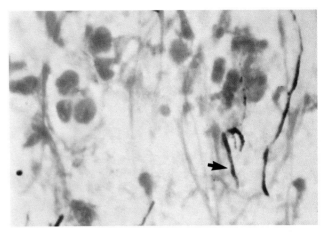

21-4. *Actinomyces israelii is a gram-positive filamentous bacterium.*

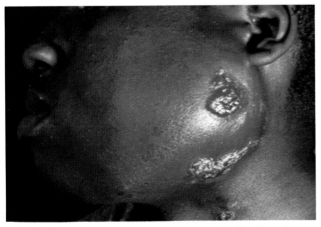

21-2. *Draining sinuses are a characteristic finding in actinomycosis.*

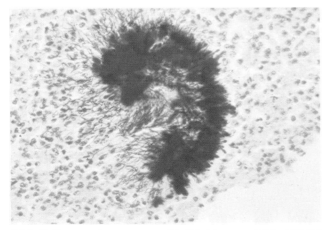

21-3. *Sulfur granules are present in this biopsy specimen from a patient with actinomycosis.*

Erythematous Patches or Nodules

Erythema nodosum

Skin

- Painful, tender, red, hot, discrete and confluent, ill-defined nodules usually occur on the anterior lower legs, but occasionally they occur on the upper extremities and face.

- Lesions are usually symmetrical.

- The color changes over time from red to brown-red to brown-yellow to brown as lesions resolve.

Pathogenesis

- This disorder represents a hypersensitivity reaction associated with a variety of infectious agents, including those causing tuberculosis, leprosy, coccidioidomycosis, histoplasmosis, psittacosis, lymphogranuloma venereum, influenza, measles, pertussis, syphilis, orf, cat-scratch disease, and beta-hemolytic streptococcal infections.

- It is also precipitated by drugs, foods, inhalants, other substances, sarcoidosis, dysproteinemias, collagen diseases, ulcerative colitis, regional enteritis, and other systemic disorders.

Clinical features

- Fever, malaise, arthralgias, and other mild systemic complaints may be present.

- Signs and symptoms of causal infecting organisms may also be present.

Differential diagnosis

- Panniculitis, bruising trauma, thrombophlebitis, erythema induratum, fat necrosis, arthropod bites, rheumatoid nodules, cellulitis, polyarteritis nodosa, nodular vasculitis.

Diagnostic tests

- Biopsy (deep wedge) shows septal panniculitis of subcutaneous tissue. (Punch-skin biopsies are usually inadequate.)

- Search elsewhere for infectious agents.

Therapy

- Eliminate cause.

- Bed rest.

- Aspirin.

- Symptomatic.

Erythema nodosum

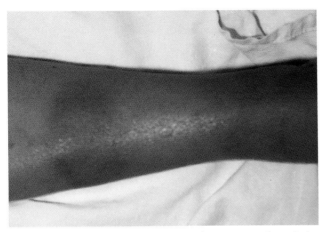

22-1. *Erythema nodosum most commonly occurs on the anterior shins.*

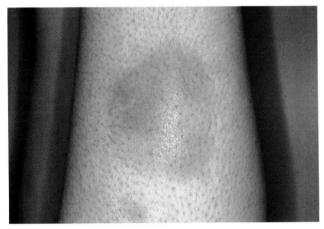

22-2. *Nodules are tender.*

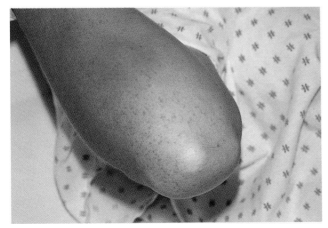

22-3. *Erythema nodosum may also occur on the arms.*

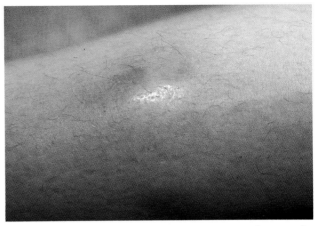

22-4. *Not all red, tender nodules on the legs are erythema nodosum. This woman had panniculitis in association with pancreatitis.*

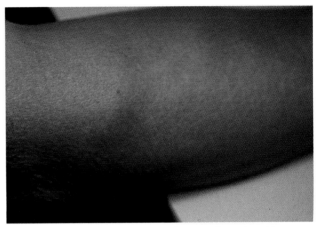

22-5. *Erythema nodosum leprosum is a manifestation of leprosy.*

Erythematous or Hypopigmented Plaques

Erythrasma

Skin
- Brown to red-brown, well-defined patches are present.
- Patches may have fine-scale or epidermal wrinkling.
- They are limited to the groin, axillae, toe webs, or breast folds.
- They may be asymptomatic or pruritic.

Pathogenesis
- Infection of stratum corneum with *Corynebacterium minutissimum* is the cause.
- Often, *Candida* species and gram-negative bacteria are also present.

Clinical features
- Findings are limited to the skin.

Differential diagnosis
- Tinea pedis or cruris, moniliasis, irritant dermatitis, allergic contact dermatitis, neurodermatitis, inverse psoriasis, gram-negative bacterial toe-web infections, intertrigo.

Diagnostic tests
- Skin fluoresces coral-red under Wood's light.
- Gram stain of epidermal scrapings shows rod-shaped, gram-positive organisms.
- Culture for corynebacteria (aerobic) is rarely necessary.

Therapy
- Oral erythromycin.
- Topical antibiotics.
- Antiperspirants.

Erythrasma

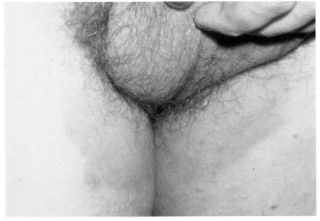

23-1. *The typical appearance of erythrasma is a brown or tan patch in an intertriginous area.*

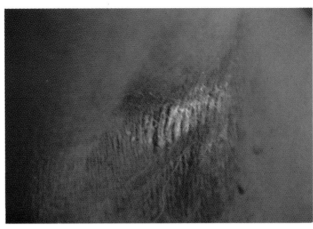

23-4. *Erythrasma fluoresces coral-red under Wood's light.*

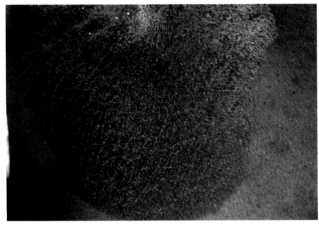

23-2. *In dark-skinned patients, the area may become intensely pigmented.*

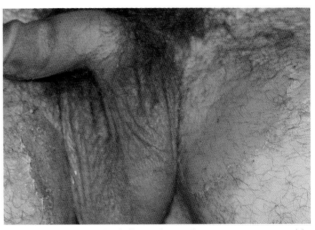

23-5. *When intensely inflamed, erythrasma may resemble cutaneous candidiasis.*

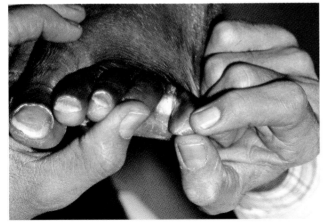

23-3. *Erythrasma involving the toe webs may be mistaken for athlete's foot.*

Erythematous or Hypopigmented Plaques

Tinea

Skin

Tinea capitis

• This infection produces irregular or nummular eczematous plaques of the scalp, with hair loss and diffuse nonscarring alopecia or broken hairs (black-dot ringworm); however, scarring may occur.

Tinea corporis

• This infection produces eczematous, mildly erythematous plaques with central clearing and elevated borders.

Tinea cruris

• This infection produces symmetric, eczematous, mildly erythematous plaques with elevated borders on upper and inner thighs and perineum; scrotum is spared, and there are no satellite lesions.

Tinea pedis and manum

• This infection produces macerated, scaling, fissured toe webs; scaling, inflammatory palms or soles; thick, friable toenails; and occasionally vesicular acute eczematous dermatitis at instep of sole.

Kerion (see section titled Pustules)

Onychomycosis (see section titled Nail Infections)

Pathogenesis

• Infection of the stratum corneum with dermatophytic fungi of the genera *Trichophyton, Epidermophyton*, or *Microsporum* is the cause.

• The presence and degree of cell-mediated immunity modifies the appearance, course, and symptomatology.

Clinical features

• Findings are limited to the skin.

• Males are affected more often than are females.

• Patient is usually in good health.

Differential diagnosis

• *Tinea capitis:* psoriasis, seborrheic dermatitis, neurodermatitis, alopecia areata, traction alopecia, impetigo, discoid lupus erythematosus.

• *Tinea corporis:* Nummular eczema, psoriasis, pityriasis rosea, granuloma annulare, erythema annulare centrifugum.

• *Tinea cruris:* Monilia, intertrigo, erythrasma, inverse psoriasis, neurodermatitis, irritant or allergic contact dermatitis.

• *Tinea pedis:* Maceration, intertrigo, pompholyx, allergic contact dermatitis from footwear, eczemas, gram-negative bacterial toe-web infections, erythrasma.

Diagnostic tests

• Dissolve scales or hair in 10% potassium hydroxide solution (KOH test) and examine microscopically for hyphae or spores.

• Fluoresce with Wood's lamp (some species).

• Culture (Mycocel or Sabouraud's agar).

• Biopsy skin with periodic acid-Schiff (PAS) stain.

Therapy

• Topical antifungal agents such as miconazole, clotrimazole, or haloprogin.

• Occasionally griseofulvin if infection refractory to topical therapy.

Tinea

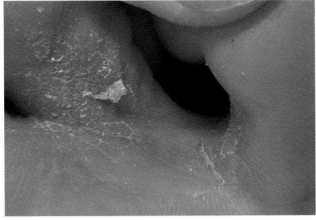

24-1. *Common athletes foot is usually associated with scaling and fissuring on the fourth-toe web.*

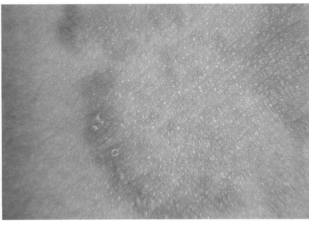

24-4. *Typically, tinea corporis assumes an annular configuration.*

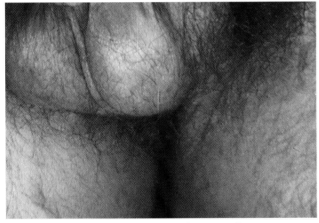

24-2. *In the groin, dermatophytes tend to spare the scrotum.*

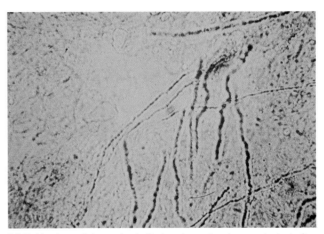

24-5. *Hyphae of dermatophytic fungi can be demonstrated after scales have been dissolved in potassium hydroxide.*

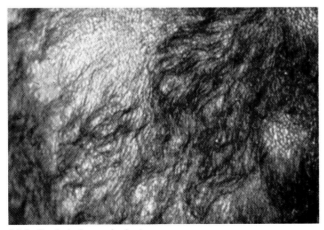

24-3. *Scalp hair may be lost.*

Erythematous or Hypopigmented Plaques

Cutaneous candidiasis

Skin
- Beefy-red, well-defined plaques, usually in body folds, with satellite plaques and pustules characterize this infection.
- Common sites are the groin, axillae, vagina, mouth, glans penis, angulus oris, and inframammary and obesity folds.
- Mucous membranes are fiery red and covered completely or partially with a creamy-white, loosely adherent coating.
- Perlèche fissures occur at angles of the mouth; perianal candidiasis mimics macerated skin.
- Chronic mucocutaneous candidiasis is a form of widespread disease with chronic, recalcitrant involvement of skin, mucous membranes, and nails.
- In candida sepsis, well-circumscribed, erythematous papulonodules, which sometimes become hemorrhagic, develop in 10% of patients.

Pathogenesis
- Infection of the stratum corneum or superficial mucosal epidermis with the yeast Candida albicans (rarely other species) is the cause.
- Inflammation is augmented by cell-mediated immune reactions.
- There is increased susceptibility in patients who have diabetes, an immunodeficiency disorder, a familial endocrinopathy syndrome, or macerated skin; in patients who are pregnant, obese, or immobile; in diapered infants; and in persons receiving antibiotics, systemic corticosteroids, or immunosuppressive drugs.

Clinical features
- Findings are usually limited to the skin.
- Systemic candidiasis is not a sequela of cutaneous candidal infection.

Differential diagnosis
- Skin: tinea cruris or pedis, intertrigo, inverse psoriasis, irritant or allergic contact dermatitis, erythrasma, maceration, acrodermatitis enteropathica.
- Mouth: lichen planus, vitamin deficiency, irritation, secondary syphilis, leukoplakia.

Diagnostic tests
- Potassium hydroxide wet mounts show spores, budding yeasts, and pseudohyphae.
- Culture on Sabouraud's or mycobiotic agar (pustule, collarette of scale, or wet area preferred); recovery of Candida does not necessarily establish etiologic role.

Therapy
- Antimonilial topical cream or solution, such as nystatin, clotrimazole, miconazole, or haloprogin.
- May combine with topical corticosteroid to lessen morbidity.
- Systemic ketoconazole if topical therapy is unsuccessful.

Cutaneous candidiasis

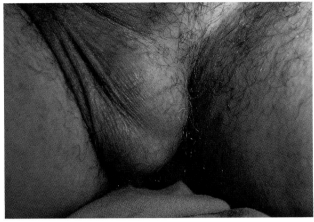

25-1. *Cutaneous Candida infections of the groin involve the scrotum.*

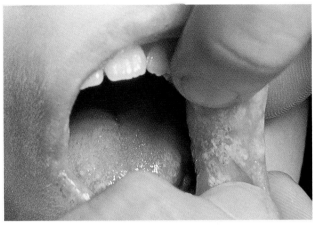

25-4. *This patient has oral candidiasis (thrush).*

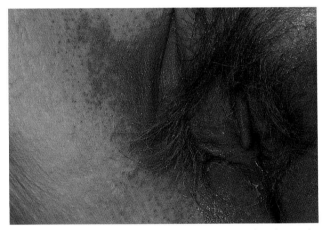

25-2. *In women, cutaneous candidiasis may involve the groin, breast folds, or other intertriginous areas.*

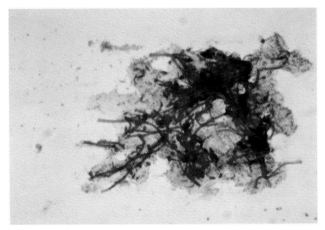

25-5. *Scrapings may show pseudohyphae.*

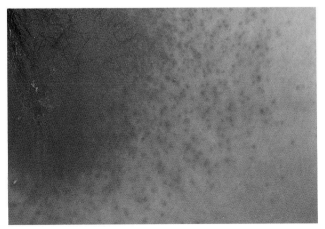

25-3. *Satellite papules or pustules often form near the edge of a beefy-red plaque.*

Erythematous or Hypopigmented Plaques

Tinea versicolor

Skin
- Slightly raised, flat-topped papules and plaques develop.
- They may be red, pink, brown, tan, or white.
- Lesions are often covered by a dust-like, nonadherent scale.
- They are located on the neck, shoulders, chest, or back (rarely on the face).
- The infection is usually asymptomatic, but sometimes mild pruritus may occur.

Pathogenesis
- The lipophilic yeast *Pityrosporium orbiculare* transforms into a mycelial organism *Malassezia furfur.*
- Predisposing conditions include Cushing's syndrome, malnutrition, and pregnancy.
- Infection is more likely to occur in summer and in humid environments.

Clinical features
- Infection can affect all ages, but teenagers and young adults are most commonly affected.
- It often recurs.
- Infected areas may not suntan.

Differential diagnosis
- Pityriasis rosea, secondary syphilis, parapsoriasis, vitiligo, pityriasis alba.

Diagnostic tests
- Potassium hydroxide (KOH) examination or methylene blue stains of scale showing hyphae and yeasts resembling spaghetti and meatballs.
- Cannot be cultured on Sabouraud's or other standard culture media.
- Wood's lamp can be used to detect clinically inapparent lesions; sometimes infected areas fluoresce slightly yellow or copper-orange.
- Scraping lesions with fingernail demonstrates dust-like scale.

Therapy
- Selenium sulfide 2.5% lotion.
- Sodium thiosulfate 25% lotion.
- Miconazole or clotrimazole cream.

Tinea versicolor

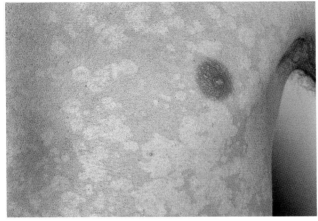

26-1. *Patients often have multiple hypopigmented macules on the chest and back.*

26-4. *Affected areas do not suntan normally.*

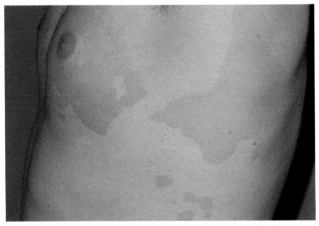

26-2. *In other stages, lesions may be salmon, pink, fawn, or brown.*

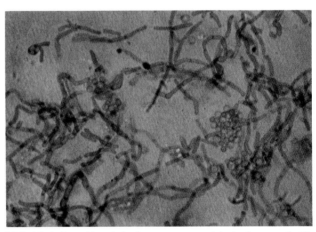

26-5. *Methylene-blue stain shows numerous interlacing spaghetti-and-meatball hyphae.*

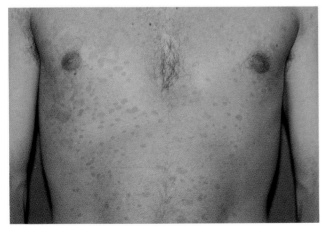

26-3. *This potentially curable disease resembles pityriasis rosea.*

Erythematous or Hypopigmented Plaques

Leprosy

Skin

Tuberculoid

- This form of disease is characterized by a few large erythematous or hypopigmented plaques with sharply demarcated edges and central clearing; the plaques are asymmetrical and anesthetic.

Borderline

- This form includes many lesions that vary in size, shape, and marginal definition; lesions tend to be symmetrical and may be hypoanesthetic.

Lepromatous

- This form is characterized by numerous papules and plaques with shiny, flat-topped, erythematous or brown surfaces; lesions usually have poorly defined edges, and satellite lesions develop outside the edge of the plaques. Often the lesions are bilaterally symmetrical, but they are not anesthetic. Multiple skin-colored nodules may occur in the ears, nose, or other sites.

Erythema nodosum leprosum (see section titled Erythematous Patches or Nodules)

Pathogenesis

- *Mycobacterium leprae* is the etiologic agent.
- The organism invades skin and peripheral nerves.
- Bacillemia is associated with involvement of the liver, spleen, and bone marrow (lepromatous leprosy).
- Classification into the three major forms of leprosy—*tuberculoid, borderline,* and *lepromatous*—depends on clinical and histopathologic findings and reflects the degree to which cell-mediated immunity develops to *M leprae.*

Clinical features

- Patients are most often immigrants from endemic areas (Far East, Mexico, Caribbean).
- *Tuberculoid:* One or more palpable, large peripheral nerves are usually found in association with skin lesions. Sensory, motor, or autonomic nerve impairment leads to paresthesias, dysesthesias, and anesthesias; neuropathy results in chronic damage and destruction of the digits and in ulcerations.
- *Borderline:* Usually widespread severe neuropathy develops.
- *Lepromatous:* Thickened facial skin (leonine facies), enlarged ears, loss of eyebrows, atrophic rhinitis (stuffy nose), eye involvement, testicular atrophy, liver disease, or lymphadenopathy develop.

Differential diagnosis

- A great imitator, leprosy mimics many skin diseases.
- Clues to diagnosis: residence in endemic country, numbness, anesthesia, enlarged nerves.

Diagnostic tests

- Punch or elliptical skin biopsy (including subcutaneous fat) with special acid-fast stains such as Fite stain (routine Ziehl-Neelsen stain may be negative).
- Bacilli abound in lepromatous leprosy but may not be seen in tuberculoid leprosy.
- Histologic picture may be characteristic, eg, histiocytic infiltration or obliteration of nerves.
- *M leprae* cannot be cultured on routine media.

Therapy

- Tuberculoid leprosy: dapsone.
- Other forms: usually dapsone plus rifampin.

Leprosy

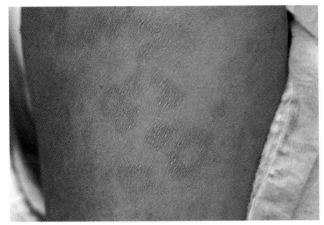

27-1. Annular erythematous plaques and hypopigmentation developed in this patient who has tuberculoid leprosy.

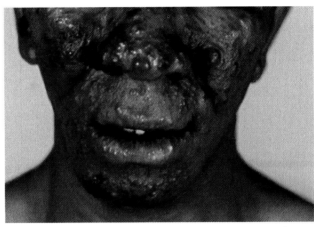

27-4. Induration of the skin in lepromatous leprosy may produce a typical leonine facies.

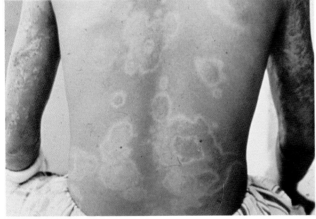

27-2. In borderline leprosy, there are many and varied lesions.

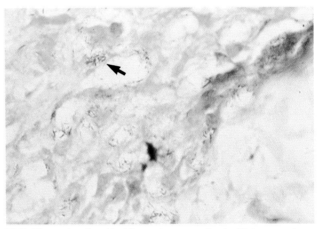

27-5. Fite stain of a skin biopsy from a patient with lepromatous leprosy shows many acid-fast bacteria.

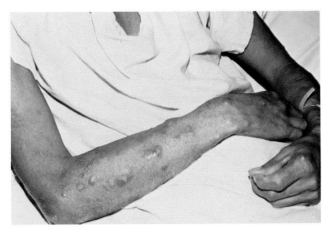

27-3. Lepromatous leprosy is characterized by numerous erythematous shiny papules and plaques.

Vesicles or Bullae

Herpes simplex virus

Skin
- Grouped vesicles arise on an erythematous base.
- Vesicles evolve to grouped pustules.
- Rupture of lesions may produce shallow ulcers covered by yellow crust.
- Lesions are usually painful, but sometimes sting or itch.

Pathogenesis
- Cytotoxic infection with herpes simplex virus (HSV) is the cause.
- It can result from primary infection or from reactivation of latent virus in nerve ganglia.

Clinical features
- Persons of any age can be affected, but primary infection usually occurs in younger children and may cause severe gingivostomatitis.
- Recurrence may be precipitated by sun, trauma, fever, menses, or other factors.
- Usual sites of recurrence are near the mouth or genitalia, but any site may be affected.

Differential diagnosis
- Herpes zoster, impetigo, chancroid, acne pustule, hand-foot-and-mouth disease, traumatic erosion.

Diagnostic tests
- Tzanck test (deroof vesicle, perform cytology on cells of blister base; herpes simplex and zoster have ballooned and multinucleated epithelial cells).
- Culture blister base or fluid for HSV.
- Serology not usually useful for recurrent herpes simplex.

Therapy
- No specific therapy available.
- Secondary bacterial infection may necessitate antibiotic therapy.
- Counsel patient on potential causes of recurrence.
- Resolution usually within ten days.
- Recurrences usually less frequent after several years.

Herpes simplex virus

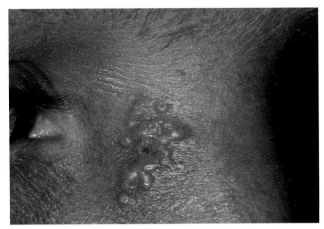

28-1. *Grouped vesicles localized on an erythematous base are typical of recurrent herpes simplex infection.*

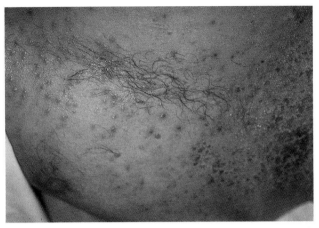

28-4. *Eczema herpeticum, a severe, more-or-less generalized eruption, usually occurs in patients who have atopic dermatitis.*

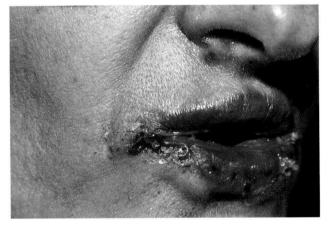

28-2. *Rupture of vesicles or pustules may produce serous or hemorrhagic crusts that mimic impetigo, as shown around this patient's mouth.*

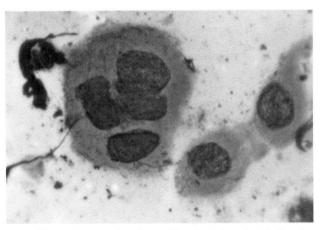

28-5. *A Tzanck smear showing multinucleated or giant ballooning epithelial cells indicates a herpesvirus infection (herpes simplex or varicella zoster).*

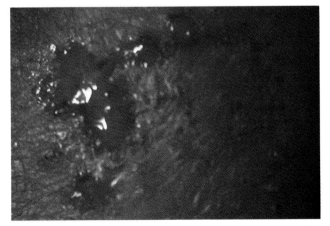

28-3. *Here is another example of herpes simplex that mimics impetigo.*

Vesicles or Bullae

Herpes zoster (shingles)

Skin
- Groups of vesicles arise on red, edematous, tender plaques that are almost always unilateral and limited to one or two contiguous dermatomes.
- The vesicles become pustules that may coalesce to form larger bullae and may become hemorrhagic.
- Crusts form after three to seven days and heal with or without scarring in about two weeks.
- The eruption is often very painful; paresthesias and pain in the affected dermatomes may precede the eruption for two to four days and persist for weeks, months, or years after the eruption clears.
- If infection is disseminated, delicate vesicles on red bases occur singly over the body surface, mimic chickenpox, and progress to pustules and then to crusts.

Pathogenesis
- A reactivation of latent herpes varicella-zoster virus in dorsal root ganglia of a partially immune individual is the cause.
- Deficient cell-mediated immunity predisposes to zoster, recurrent zoster, and disseminated zoster.
- Cutaneous dissemination with a few scattered vesicles outside the dermatome occurs in 15% of patients.
- Severe generalized dissemination with hundreds of scattered lesions may occur in patients with impaired immunity due to old age, malignancy, Hodgkin's disease, lymphatic leukemia, therapeutic immunosuppression, or immunodeficiency.
- Herpes zoster is a communicable disease (it can cause chickenpox in nonimmune contacts).

Clinical features
- Persons of any age can be affected, but most commonly persons are 50 to 80 years old.
- Most patients feel otherwise well, but pain may be disabling.
- Sacral zoster may lead to acute urinary retention.
- Ophthalmic zoster (ophthalmic branch of trigeminal nerve) may lead to conjunctivitis, keratitis, iridocyclitis, and paralysis of extraocular muscles.
- Rarely, motor paralysis (eg, of extremity, diaphragm, eye muscles, facial muscles) occurs.
- Complications include cutaneous bacterial superinfection and postherpetic neuralgia (rare in persons less than 40 years old); dissemination (rare even in immunodeficient hosts) may lead to encephalomyelitis, pneumonitis, or gastrointestinal tract involvement.

Differential diagnosis
- Herpes simplex, occasionally impetigo, varicella, localized bullous pemphigoid, cellulitis.
- Pain alone: trigeminal neuralgia, pleurisy, myocardial infarction, acute abdomen, herniated disc syndrome.
- Paralysis alone: Bell's palsy, overflow incontinence, constipation, intracranial aneurysm.

Diagnostic tests
- Tzanck smear of base of vesicle may show giant, ballooned, and multinucleated epithelial cells (see section titled Herpes Simplex).
- Culture to isolate varicella-zoster virus.
- Serology: fourfold rise in antibody titer.

Therapy
- Symptomatic, analgesics.
- Shake lotions or wet compresses.
- Systemic corticosteroids given early in patients over 60 years old may decrease incidence of postherpetic neuralgia.
- Systemic vidarabine early (immunosuppressed patients).
- Isolation of hospitalized patients.

Herpes zoster (shingles)

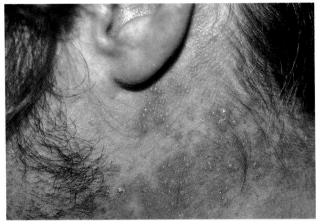

29-1. *In herpes zoster, grouped vesicles arise on painful erythematous plaques.*

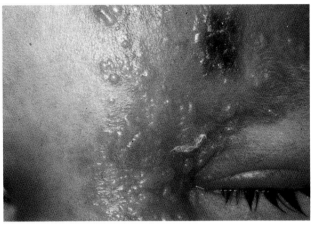

29-4. *Involvement of the dermatome supplied by the ophthalmic branch of the trigeminal nerve may lead to herpes keratitis.*

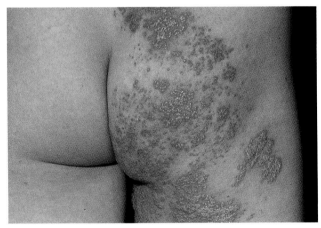

29-2. *The distribution follows dermatomes.*

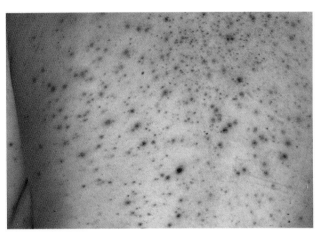

29-5. *Disseminated herpes zoster resembles varicella.*

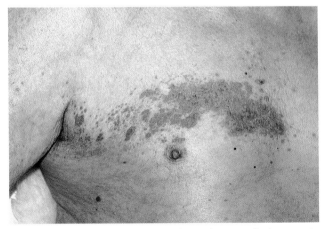

29-3. *Later, vesicles become pustules and eventually they crust.*

Vesicles or Bullae

Varicella (chickenpox)

Skin

- Crops of vesicles 2 to 4 mm in diameter progress rapidly from red macules to papules to pustules to crusts.
- A few or many lesions in all stages of development may be present simultaneously.
- Vesicles are delicate ("dewdrops on rose petals").
- A centripetal pattern develops; more lesions are present on the trunk than on the extremities.
- Pruritus is variable.

Pathogenesis

- Primary viremia of varicella-zoster virus is the cause.
- Lesions of the skin and mucous membranes (including gastrointestinal, respiratory, and urinary tracts) may develop.
- Epidemic transmission occurs, usually by respiratory droplets.

Clinical features

- Ninety percent of affected persons are children.
- Young children usually seem well.
- Older children and adults commonly have fever, headache, malaise, myalgias, and prolonged convalescence.
- Complications are most common in neonates, adults, immunosuppressed persons, and persons who have leukemia; complications include varicella bullosum, impetigo, varicella pneumonia, encephalitis, and disseminated intravascular coagulation (purpura fulminans).

Differential diagnosis

- Disseminated herpes zoster, smallpox (now extinct), impetigo, dermatitis herpetiformis, pityriasis lichenoides et varioliformis acuta, folliculitis.

Diagnostic tests

- Usually a clinical diagnosis.
- Tzanck smear (Giemsa's stain of cells of vesicle base) shows multinucleated and giant cells (see section titled Herpes Simplex).
- Culture of skin lesions.
- Serology: fourfold rise in antibody titer.

Therapy

- Symptomatic.
- Systemic antibiotics for significant bacterial superinfection.

Varicella (chickenpox)

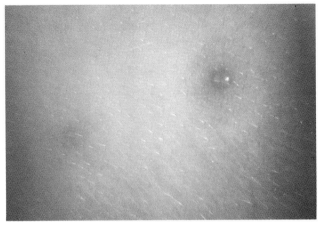

30-1. *The vesicle of varicella has been likened to a dewdrop on a rose petal.*

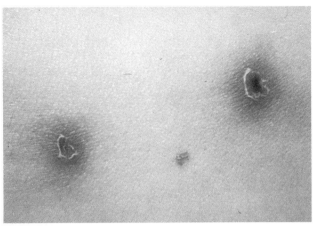

30-4. *Finally, the lesions crust.*

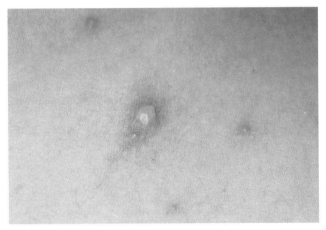

30-2. *Vesicles soon become pustules.*

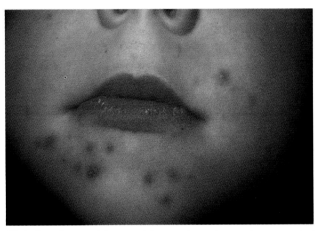

30-5. *Papules, vesicles, pustules, and crusts may be present at the same time.*

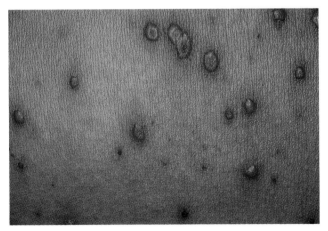

30-3. *Umbilication occurs in the late pustular stage.*

Vesicles or Bullae

Hand-foot-and-mouth disease

Skin
- The mouth is usually affected first with multiple, small fragile vesicles, especially on the tongue, hard palate, buccal mucosa, lips, and pharynx.
- Rupture of vesicles produces shallow ulcers.
- Multiple round or oval vesicles, 2 to 10 mm in diameter, surrounded by red areolae, arise on the sides of fingers and toes and on both sides of the hands and feet.
- Orientation of oval vesicles is along skin lines.
- Vesicles become flaccid or they rupture; then they crust and resolve in seven to ten days.
- Rarely, disseminated vesicles or maculopapules develop.

Pathogenesis
- Infection with an enterovirus of the picorna-virus group, usually coxsackie A16 or A5, but also A9, A10, B2, or B7, is the cause.

Clinical features
- Infection usually occurs in children and is often epidemic.
- Low-grade fever, malaise, arthralgias, and sore throat or mouth may be present.
- Patient may feel rather well.
- Recovery after seven to ten days is likely.
- Rarely, aseptic meningitis, paralytic disease, or myocarditis occurs.

Differential diagnosis
- Herpes simplex, herpangina, aphthous stomatitis, herpetiform ulcers of the mouth, pompholyx, allergic contact dermatitis, erythema multiforme, pemphigus.

Diagnostic tests
- Usually a clinical diagnosis.
- If necessary, culture vesicle fluid, throat smear, and stool specimen.
- Serial serologic tests (neutralizing and complement-fixing antibodies).

Therapy
- No specific therapy.
- Topical anesthetics for oral lesions.

Hand-foot-and-mouth disease

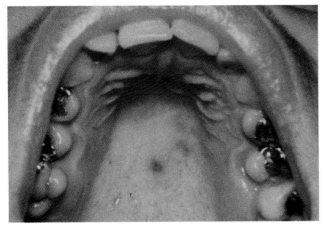

31-1. *Multiple ulcers in the mouth are, by themselves, nonspecific.*

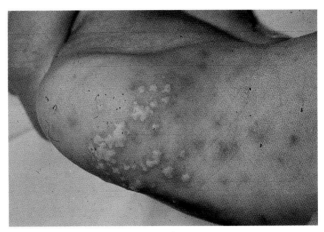

31-4. *Vesicles may become pustules.*

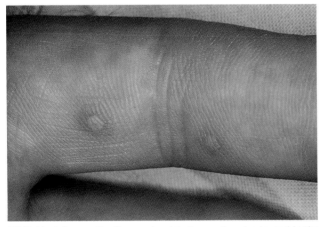

31-2. *Vesicles on the fingers tend to be oval and oriented in the direction of skin markings.*

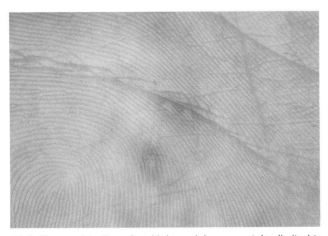

31-3. *The combination of multiple vesicles or pustules limited to the hands and feet in a patient who has mouth ulcers is both typical and virtually diagnostic.*

Vesicles or Bullae

Staphylococcal scalded skin syndrome (SSSS)

Skin
- A scarlatiniform rash is present early, and the skin may be tender.
- Exfoliation develops, with separation of sheets of skin (red denuded base).
- Widespread, flaccid, clear, large bullae may develop.
- Lateral traction on affected skin may cause peeling (positive Nikolsky sign).

Pathogenesis
- In the presence of infection caused by phage group II *Staphylococcus aureus,* an exfoliative toxin may be produced, and the toxin causes the disease.
- The toxin causes the epidermal cells to separate from each other and produces a characteristic cleavage plane high in the epidermis.

Clinical features
- Usually infants or young children are affected; adults are rarely affected, but those who are often have depressed immune function or renal failure.
- Abrupt onset with fever and skin tenderness may occur.
- The site of infection is usually distant from the lesions.

Differential diagnosis
- Morphologically indistinguishable from toxic epidermal necrolysis (TEN), which is a pathogenically unrelated disease caused by drugs, viral infections, or lymphoma.
- Scarlet fever; thermal scald.

Diagnostic tests
- Biopsy through bulla (look for characteristic cleavage plane in upper epidermis).
- Cultures (blood, abscesses, and so forth), phage-typing of *S aureus* isolates.

Therapy
- Penicillinase-resistant penicillin, intravenously.
- Fluid replacement.
- Local care with cool saline compresses.
- Skin usually heals in two weeks.

Staphylococcal scalded skin syndrome (SSSS)

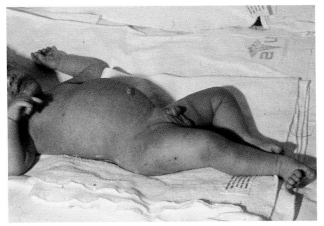

32-1. *In children, the first skin manifestation of SSSS is a generalized erythema.*

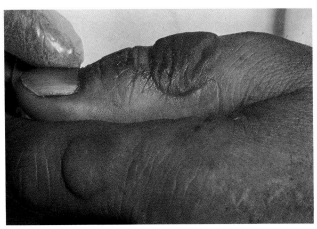

32-4. *When bullae occur, they are typically flaccid.*

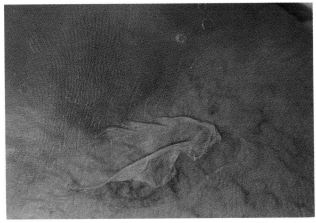

32-2. *The epidermis may peel off in sheets, resembling a burn injury.*

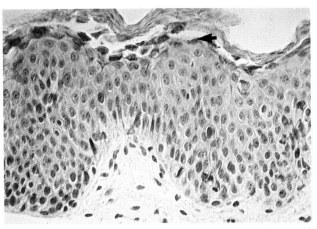

32-5. *The cleavage plane in SSSS is high in the epidermis (arrow) and can be distinguished from drug-induced toxic epidermal necrolysis by biopsy.*

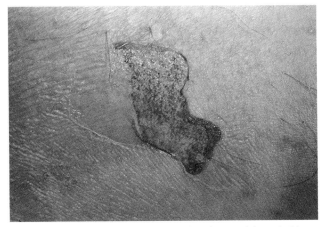

32-3. *Following separation of the epidermis, a red denuded base is seen.*

Pustules

Acne

Skin

- Open or closed comedones, inflammatory papules, pustules, and nodules characterize acne.
- Lesions are usually limited to the face, upper chest, and back.
- Scars from previous lesions may be present.

Pathogenesis

- Acne is an inflammatory disease of the pilosebaceous unit and occurs primarily in adolescence.
- The anaerobic bacterium *Propionibacterium acnes* may play a role by hydrolizing fats to fatty acids.
- Dyskeratosis at the follicular orifice may lead to blockage of the duct, which leads to duct rupture and subsequent liberation of duct contents into surrounding tissue.
- Inflammation follows duct rupture and is primarily a foreign-body response.
- Acne can be exacerbated by drugs (steroids, androgens, oral contraceptives, halogens, anticonvulsants, lithium, vitamin B_{12}, antituberculous drugs, and others), adrenal or ovarian dysfunction, external oils and cosmetics, trauma, and other factors.

Clinical features

- Most individuals are in good health.
- Acne fulminans is associated with fever, malaise, and arthralgias.

Differential diagnosis

- Acneiform drug eruption, rosacea, folliculitis, milia, pyoderma faciale, perioral dermatitis, pseudofolliculitis barbae, sycosis barbae, chloracne.

Diagnostic tests

- Almost always a clinical diagnosis.

Therapy

- Antibiotics (topical or systemic).
- Keratolytics.
- Soaps and cleansing.
- Retinoic acid.

Acne

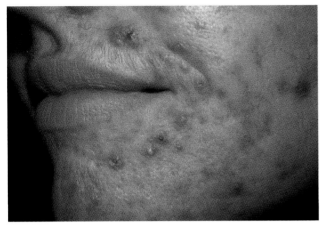

33-1. *Inflammatory papules and pustules are present on the face, chest, and back.*

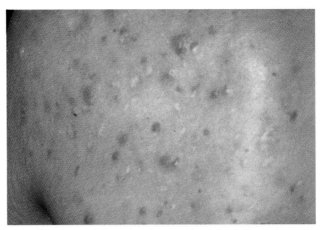

33-4. *Acne conglobata is characterized by inflamed, cystic nodules.*

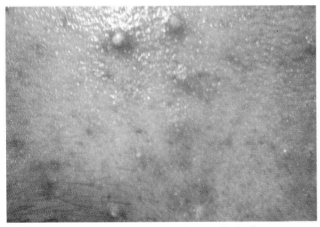

33-2. *The skin in the area of the pustules may look oily.*

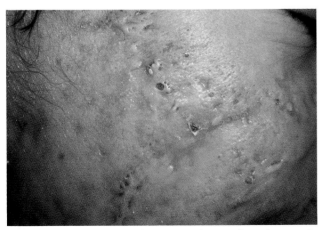

33-3. *Open comedones and scars are the prominent features in this patient.*

Pustules

Folliculitis

Skin

- Pinhead-sized erythematous papules often topped by superficial pustules located at follicular orifices characterize this infection.

- Each pustule may be pierced by a hair.

- Lesions may be single or multiple and may occur on any hair-bearing site, such as the thighs.

- On the scalp, lesions may scar and cause permanent hair loss.

- Sycosis barbae: deep folliculitis of bearded skin is often chronic.

Pathogenesis

- The upper portion of hair follicles becomes infected by *Staphylococcus aureus.*

- Occasionally, *Pseudomonas aeruginosa* (from swimming pools or whirlpools), pityrosporium yeasts, anaerobic bacteria, diphtheroids, or other bacteria may be pathogenic.

- Folliculitis may also be caused by contact with chemicals or by mechanical trauma, in which case pustules are often sterile.

Clinical features

- Findings are limited to the skin.

Differential diagnosis

- Pseudofolliculitis barbae, bites, keratosis pilaris, lichen niditis, subcorneal pustular dermatosis, acne vulgaris, chloracne, foreign-body reaction, acneiform drug reaction, milia, miliaria pustulosa, tinea corporis.

Diagnostic tests

- Usually a clinical diagnosis.

- Stain of pustule contents may show gram-positive cocci, and culture may yield *S aureus.*

Therapy

- Topical modalities (eg, benzoyl peroxide gels, keratolytics).

- Systemic antibiotics for severe cases.

Folliculitis

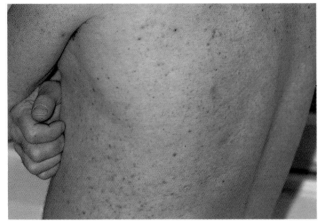

34-1. *Folliculitis is characterized by scattered, small papules and pustules.*

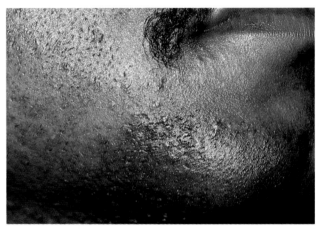

34-4. *Pseudofolliculitis mimics bacterial folliculitis but is caused by ingrown hairs.*

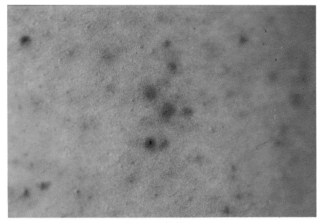

34-2. *Each lesion occurs in a hair follicle.*

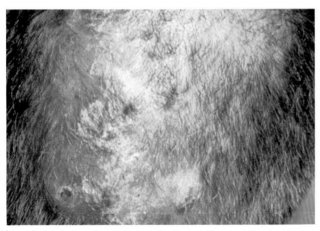

34-3. *In folliculitis decalvans, hair follicles are destroyed.*

Pustules

Hidradenitis suppurativa

Skin
- This infection usually produces multiple, inflamed, tender cysts of axillary skin or perianal skin or both.
- A tender nodule progresses to an abscess that leads to a draining abscess and often to chronically draining sinuses and scarring.
- Draining material is purulent or seropurulent.
- Complications include open sinuses of the axillary vault, lymphedema of the extremity, perianal fistulae, and abscesses of the penis.

Pathogenesis
- An infection of apocrine ducts, usually with *Staphylococcus aureus*, is the cause, but it may involve streptococci and gram-negative aerobes and anaerobes.
- Poral occlusion leads to dilatation of apocrine ducts, infection, infiltration with polymorphonuclear leukocytes, rupture of duct, chronic inflammation and suppuration, and fibrosis and sinus tract formation.
- Obese individuals are predisposed.

Clinical features
- Most patients are 15 to 40 years old.
- Patients are usually in good health.
- Associated acne conglobata and folliculitis of the head may occur.

Differential diagnosis
- Abscess, furuncle, carbuncle, infected cyst, perianal fistulae of other causes, draining lymph nodes (seen in tularemia, tuberculosis, lymphogranuloma venereum, actinomycosis, granuloma inguinale, cat scratch disease, amebiasis, and plague).

Diagnostic tests
- Clinical diagnosis.
- Culture (useful as guide to antibiotic selection).

Therapy
- Systemic antibiotics.
- Intralesional corticosteroids.
- Intermittent warm, wet compresses.
- Cleansing and topical antibiotics.
- Surgical excision of axillary vault or affected areas, or exteriorization of fistulae in longstanding cases.
- Discontinuation of use of antiperspirants.
- Weight reduction.

Hidradenitis suppurativa

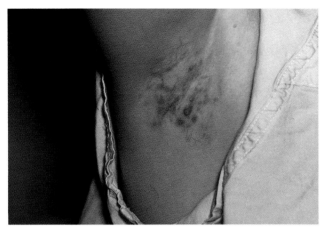

35-1. *Multiple abscesses in the axilla are more likely to be hidradenitis suppurativa than furuncles.*

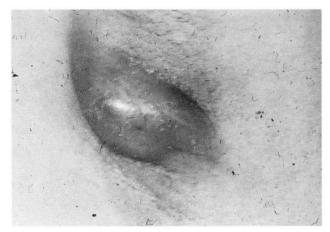

35-2. *Sometimes the abscesses are quite large.*

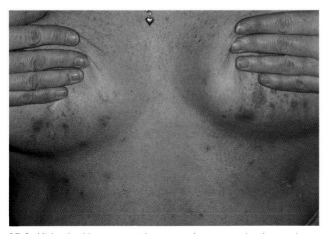

35-3. *Hidradenitis suppurativa can also occur in the groin or breast area.*

Pustules

Furuncles

Skin

- Infection produces small tender nodules or larger fluctuant abscesses.
- Lesions may be single (furuncle), multiple and contiguous (carbuncle), or multiple and recurrent (furunculosis).
- Lesions often rupture spontaneously and drain purulent material.
- Lesions can occur anywhere on hair-bearing skin, especially buttocks, thighs, and abdomen.
- Later, nodules become violaceous and heal, often with depressed scars.

Pathogenesis

- Hair follicles become infected, usually with *Staphylococcus aureus* but also with anaerobes or gram-negative aerobes or both, depending on body location.
- Usually there is no detectable abnormality of immune function, but in severe or recurrent cases, an immuno-deficiency state should be considered.
- Predisposed individuals are those who are obese or diabetic or who have poor hygiene.

Clinical features

- Patients are usually in good health.
- Most patients are 15 to 40 years old.

Differential diagnosis

- Folliculitis, acne, hidradenitis suppurativa, iododerma, infected cyst, pilonidal cyst, perirectal abscess.

Diagnostic tests

- Clinical diagnosis.
- Culture (as a guide to antibiotic selection).

Therapy

- Incision and drainage.
- Systemic antibiotics for severe or recurrent cases.
- Warm, wet compresses.

Furuncles

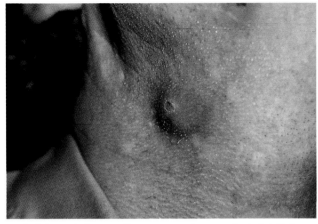

36-1. *A furuncle is a small cutaneous abscess of a hair follicle.*

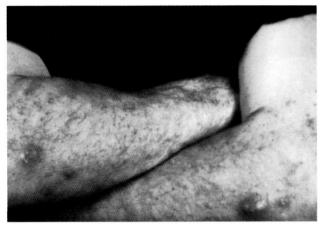

36-2. *Lesions may be multiple or recurrent, or both (furunculosis).*

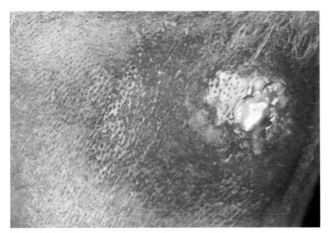

36-3. *Multiple and contiguous abscesses form a carbuncle.*

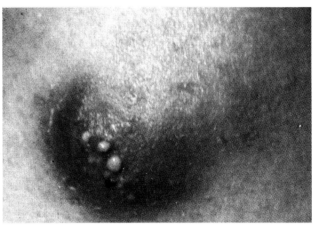

36-4. *Pus may drain spontaneously or may be expressed from a mature furuncle.*

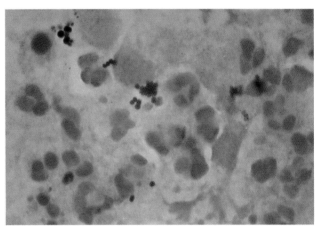

36-5. *Gram-positive cocci in clusters are often seen in smears of aspirated pus.*

Pustules

Kerion

Skin

- A painful, rounded, boggy, erythematous, carbuncle-like tumor develops, usually in scalp or beard; it is often suppurating.
- Hair falls out of skin over the lesion, or it can easily be removed by slight traction.
- The surface is studded with pinhead-sized pustules, gaping follicular orifices, pus, or yellow crust.

Pathogenesis

- Infection of hair follicles, usually with *Trichophyton verrucosum* but sometimes other species of *Trichophyton* or *Microsporum* or other fungi, is the cause.
- Inflammatory reaction is augmented by the presence of cell-mediated immunity.

Clinical features

- Infection often occurs in farmers or children.
- Patients are usually in good health.
- Fever and regional lymphadenopathy occur in some cases.

Differential diagnosis

- Scalp abscess, carbuncle, iododerma.

Diagnostic tests

- Usually a clinical diagnosis.
- Potassium hydroxide (KOH) examination of plucked hair may show spores.
- Culture for dermatophytes.
- Most fungi that cause kerions do *not* fluoresce under Wood's light.

Therapy

- Infection may be self-limited.
- Griseofulvin.
- Systemic antibiotics and corticosteroids in some patients.
- Intermittent wet compresses.
- Incision and drainage not recommended.

Kerion

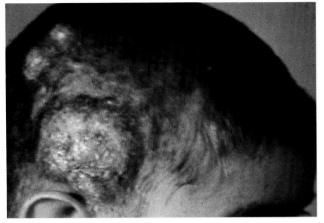

37-1. *A kerion is a boggy, rounded, carbuncle-like tumor, usually on the scalp.*

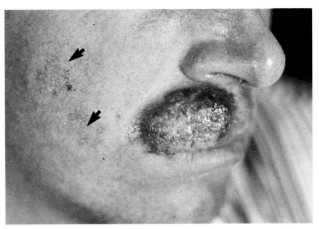

37-4. *This kerion is associated with at least two patches of tinea faciale (arrows).*

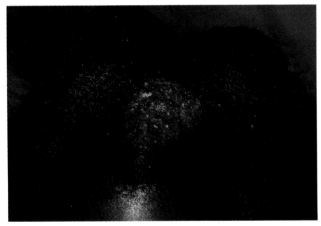

37-2. *Overlying hair is frequently lost.*

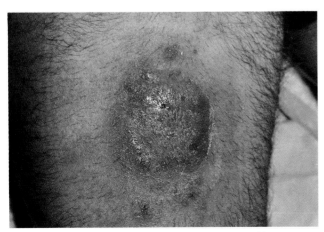

37-3. *Kerions can occur anywhere on hair-bearing skin.*

Pustules

Herpetic whitlow

Skin
- This infection is characterized by intense itching or pain and grouped vesicles that coalesce, spread, and become pustular.
- Most lesions are on the fingers near the fingernails, often on the dominant hand.

Pathogenesis
- This primary infection of the skin of the fingers is caused by *herpes simplex virus.*
- It is usually introduced by direct contact of the skin with active herpes infection.
- In immunosuppressed persons, it may be introduced by autoinoculation from herpes labialis.
- Nurses, dentists, and doctors are especially predisposed, particularly those contacting oral mucosae and tracheotomy stomae.

Clinical features
- Severe pain and occasional headache or malaise may occur.
- Regional lymphadenopathy may also develop.

Differential diagnosis
- Acute bacterial paronychia, foreign-body reaction, bacterial abscess, milker's nodule, orf.

Diagnostic tests
- Tzanck smear of cells at base of vesicles shows ballooned giant cells, often multinucleated (see section titled Herpes Simplex Virus).
- Culture (base or vesicle fluid).

Therapy
- Symptomatic.
- Soaks, analgesics.

Herpetic whitlow

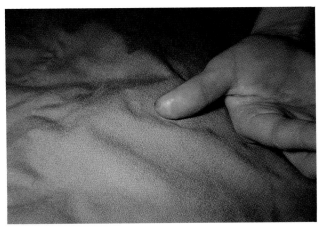

38-1. *Painful, deep-seated, grouped pustules occur on fingertips.*

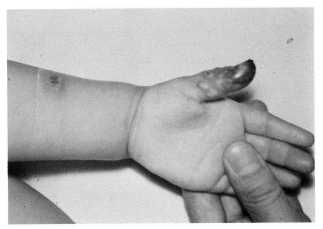

38-4. *Thumbsuckers with herpetic gingivostomatitis may develop herpetic whitlows.*

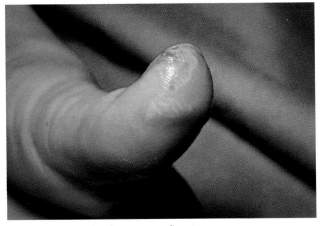

38-2. *Later, pustules become confluent.*

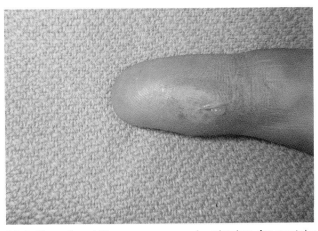

38-3. *Herpetic whitlows are commonly mistaken for pustular bacterial lesions and are unnecessarily incised.*

Pustules

Ecthyma contagiosum (orf)

Skin

- A red-to-purple, tender papule develops into a larger hemorrhagic pustule that may become an umbilicated pustule. The pustule may rupture and leave an ulcerated nodule with gray-white crust.
- Lesions may be single or multiple; they usually occur on exposed surfaces (usually hands).
- A transient erythematous rash may appear on the trunk during the second week of illness.
- Erythema multiforme may occur after two weeks.

Pathogenesis

- Orf virus, a poxvirus of sheep, accidentally infects humans at the site of a bite or abrasion.

Clinical features

- Affected persons (farmers, butchers, and veterinarians most often) have contacted sheep, especially newborn lambs.
- Low-grade fever and regional lymphadenitis may be present.

Differential diagnosis

- Milker's nodule, anthrax, tularemia, pyogenic granuloma, squamous cell carcinoma, herpetic whitlow.

Diagnostic tests

- Usually a clinical diagnosis.
- Viral culture.
- Electron microscopy shows large ovoid virus particles.

Therapy

- Symptomatic; spontaneous healing in three to six weeks.

Ecthyma contagiosum (orf)

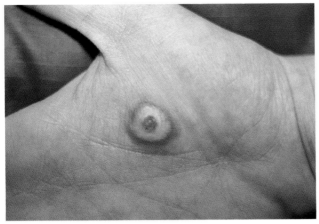

39-1. *Relatively early lesions of orf are large pustules on a red base.*

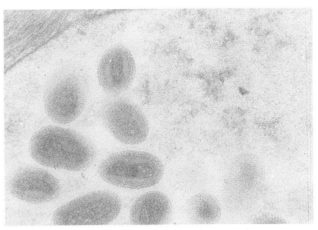

39-4. *Orf virus can be demonstrated by electron microscopy.*

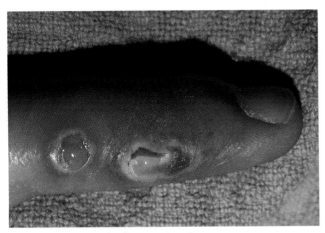

39-2. *Here the pustules have ruptured.*

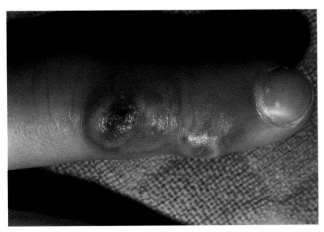

39-3. *Lesions most commonly occur on the fingers of sheep handlers.*

Pustules

Milker's nodule

Skin

- Usually a solitary macule on a finger, hand, or wrist develops into a papule 1 to 2 cm in diameter and then progresses to a red-to-violet vesiconodule. Finally, central umbilication and crusting develop. The characteristic lesion has a central crust, a surrounding white vesicopustule, and an erythematous base. The nodule resolves in two to three weeks.

Pathogenesis

- Infection of the skin by a poxvirus (paravaccinia virus) is the cause.
- It is transmitted to humans by direct contact with infected cattle (pseudocowpox) or by contact with another infected human.

Clinical features

- Farmers and butchers are predisposed.
- Patients are usually in good health.
- Occasionally, lymphangitis or regional lymphadenopathy is present.

Differential diagnosis

- Orf, cowpox, herpetic whitlow, furuncle, pyoderma, anthrax, tularemia, tuberculosis verrucosis cutis, atypical mycobacterial infection, sporotrichosis, chancre of syphilis, pyogenic granuloma, vaccinia.

Diagnostic tests

- Usually a clinical diagnosis.
- Electron microscopy reveals characteristic brick-shaped virus.
- Culture.

Therapy

- Symptomatic.
- Wet compresses.

Milker's nodule

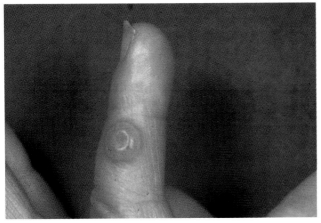

40-1. *Early milker's nodule is a red-to-violet lesion that appears almost vesicular.*

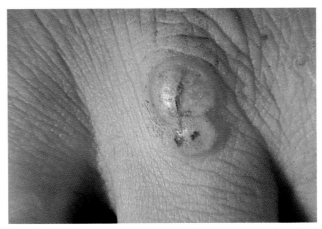

40-4. *Milker's nodules most commonly occur on the hands of dairy farmers.*

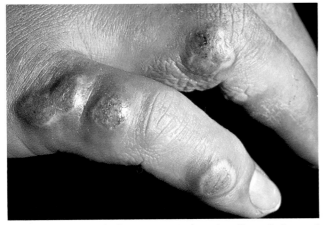

40-2. *Typical target lesions are central crusts with encircling red and white rings.*

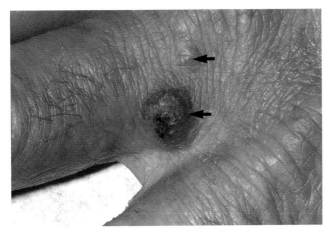

40-3. *Other lesions are crusted nodules. Note the presence of new satellite papules (arrows).*

Petechiae, Purpura, or Ecchymoses

Rocky Mountain spotted fever

Skin

- A rash appears usually between the second and sixth days of illness, but it is occasionally absent, delayed, or undetected, especially in blacks.
- Initially, small erythematous macules that blanch on pressure become maculopapular, with development of petechiae, purpura, and ecchymoses.
- The rash first appears on wrists and ankles, then spreads to the extremities and trunk.
- The palms and soles are almost always involved.
- Small areas of necrosis (fingers, toes, earlobes, scrotum, vulva) may occur.

Pathogenesis

- *Rickettsia rickettsii,* transmitted by ticks (wood tick, dog tick, or Lone Star tick), is the cause.
- The organisms multiply within endothelial cells of small blood vessels, leading to leakage and thrombosis.

Clinical features

- Two thirds of patients are less than 15 years old.
- The disease is most common in the Southeastern United States (less than 5% of cases occur in the Rocky Mountain area).
- It is largely a seasonal disease (spring and summer).
- Onset is gradual or abrupt.
- Fever (high, spiking), severe headache, toxicity, confusion, and myalgia commonly occur.
- Stiff neck, conjunctival suffusion, muscle tenderness, and splenomegaly may also be present.
- Other complications include disseminated intravascular coagulation, renal failure, pulmonary edema (adult respiratory distress syndrome), or pneumonia (late).

Differential diagnosis

- Meningococcemia, rubeola, atypical measles, typhoid fever, leptospirosis, infectious mononucleosis, dengue, other rickettsial diseases.

Diagnostic tests

- Biopsy skin lesion for Rickettsia in small blood vessels (positive specific immunofluorescence antibody staining by day four or five of the illness).
- Serologic tests (Weil-Felix test and complement fixation test): single high titer or fourfold titer change (usually takes eight to ten days; therefore, of limited clinical value).
- Culture (usually not practical and potentially dangerous to laboratory personnel).

Therapy

- 20% mortality if untreated—therapy must be initiated before diagnosis is established.
- Chloramphenicol or tetracycline.

Rocky Mountain spotted fever

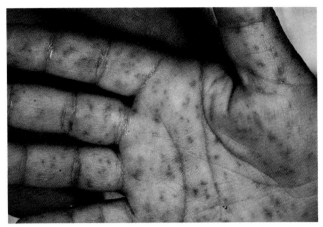

41-1. *Palms and soles are almost always involved.*

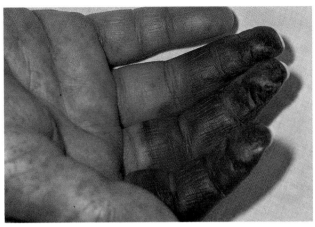

41-4. *Progression to gangrene is rare.*

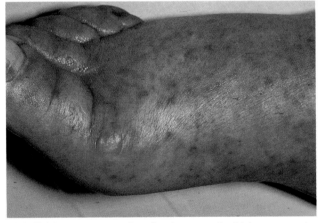

41-2. *Erythematous macules often have a petechial component.*

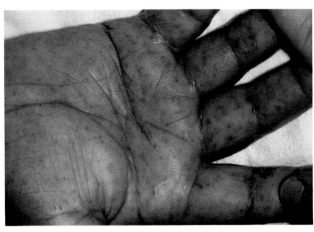

41-5. *Among other diseases characterized by hemorrhagic lesions on the palms and soles are atypical measles, measles, meningococcemia, and dengue.*

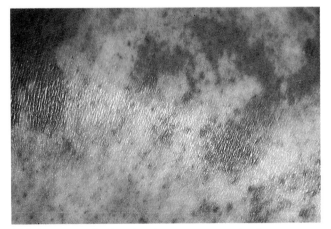

41-3. *In some patients, extensive purpura may develop.*

Petechiae, Purpura, or Ecchymoses

Meningococcemia

Skin

Acute meningococcemia

- Erythematous macules, petechiae, purpura, and ecchymosis commonly begin on trunk and legs in areas where pressure is applied.
- Confluence of petechial and purpuric lesions results in hemorrhagic patches, often with central necrosis.

Chronic meningococcemia

- Variability is a hallmark; erythematous maculopapular, petechial, nodular, or vesiculopapular lesions may be present.
- At time of fever, rash occurs in crops on extremities, especially around joints.

Pathogenesis

- *Neisseria meningitidis* bacteremia produces acute vasculitis or local Shwartzman-like reaction, with purpura.
- Disseminated intravascular coagulation may develop.
- Adrenal hemorrhage (Waterhouse-Friderichsen syndrome) may occur.
- Complement deficiency (C5, C6, C7, or C8) is present in some patients.

Clinical features

- *Acute meningococcemia:* Patients may have fever, malaise, weakness, headache, and hypotension.
- Meningeal signs or abnormal mental status or both may be present in patients with meningitis. Myocarditis or pericarditis may be present; endocarditis is rare.
- *Chronic meningococcemia:* Episodes of fever, arthralgias, anorexia, headache, and rash recur over several months.

Differential diagnosis

- Hemorrhagic rashes or petechial rashes or both: Rocky Mountain spotted fever, other bacterial infections (gonococcal, pneumococcal, staphylococcal, group A streptococcal, clostridial, gram-negative bacteremia, plague, rat-bite fever), infective endocarditis.
- Viral infections: rubeola, varicella, ECHO* 9 or 16, Colorado tick fever, acute hemorrhagic fevers (dengue, yellow fever, Korean hemorrhagic fevers, Machupo virus, Lassa fever virus).
- Schönlein-Henoch purpura, hypersensitivity vasculitis.
- Purpura fulminans, disseminated intravascular coagulation from other causes.

Diagnostic tests

- Lumbar puncture with cerebrospinal fluid (CSF) analysis, including Gram stain (purulent CSF and purpura or ecchymoses virtually diagnostic).
- Cultures (blood, CSF).
- Occasionally gram-negative diplococci are seen on smears of tissue fluid from skin in acute meningococcemia.

Therapy

- Supportive care.
- Penicillin G.
- Steroids in adrenal insufficiency.

*ECHO virus: enterocytopathogenic human orphan virus.

Meningococcemia

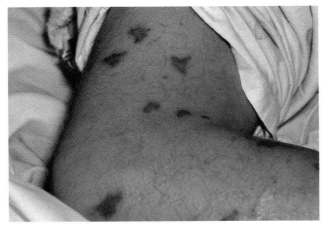

42-1. *These are relatively early purpuric lesions of meningococcemia.*

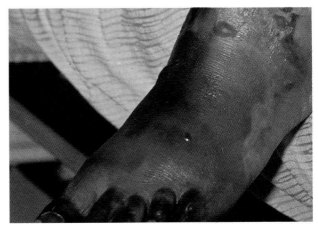

42-4. *Vasculitis may result in peripheral gangrene.*

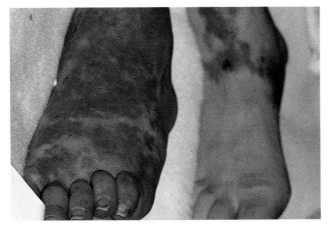

42-2. *Purpura becomes confluent to create extensive hemorrhagic patches.*

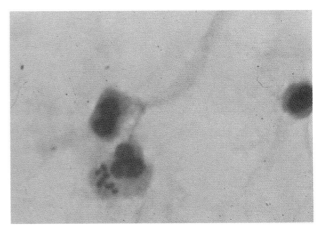

42-5. *The presence of gram-negative diplococci in the cerebrospinal fluid is virtually diagnostic.*

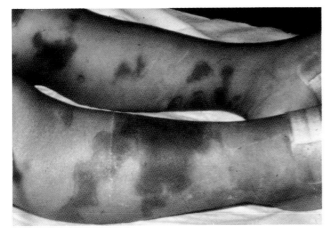

42-3. *Hemorrhagic patches may become necrotic.*

Petechiae, Purpura, or Ecchymoses

Disseminated gonococcal infection

Skin
- Lesions begin as tiny red papules or petechiae and may evolve into purpuric pustules, vesicles, or bullae.
- Pustules on an erythematous or hemorrhagic base are characteristic.
- Few lesions (from five to 40) are present.
- Lesions are scattered over distal extremities (sparing the face and trunk), and frequently they are painful.

Pathogenesis
- *Neisseria gonorrhoeae* disseminates from an anogenital or pharyngeal site (bacteremic stage), with invasion of skin.
- Direct toxic (endotoxin) effect of gonococcus or immune complex vasculitis or both cause tissue injury.

Clinical features
- Infection is most common in women who have multiple sexual partners; dissemination often occurs during menstruation.
- The primary anogenital gonococcal infection is usually asymptomatic.
- Polyarthralgias, tenosynovitis, or monoarticular arthritis (dermatitis-arthritis syndrome) may be present.
- Fever, chills, and leukocytosis commonly occur.
- Abnormalities are seen in liver function test results.
- Rarely, meningitis, myocarditis, pericarditis, and endocarditis occur.

Differential diagnosis
- Reiter's syndrome, other septic arthritis, meningococcemia, infective endocarditis, acute rheumatoid arthritis, systemic lupus erythematosus.

Diagnostic tests
- Culture: blood (usually positive early), synovial fluid, rectal, genital, pharyngeal.
- Gram stain and culture of skin lesions may be positive.
- Specific immunofluorescent antibody staining of skin or synovial fluid usually reveals organisms.

Therapy
- Intravenous penicillin G (or high-dose ampicillin or amoxicillin).

Disseminated gonococcal infection

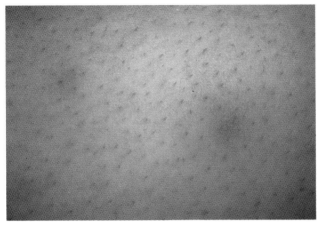

43-1. *Early lesions are nondiagnostic erythematous macules.*

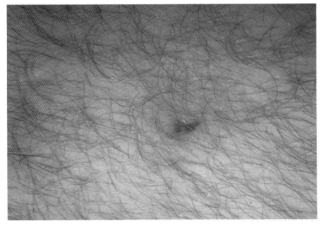

43-2. *A typical lesion is a hemorrhagic pustule on an erythematous base.*

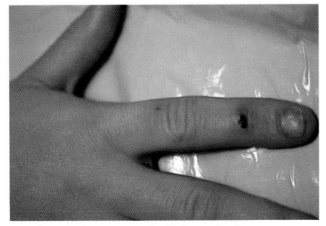

43-3. *Some lesions are more frankly hemorrhagic.*

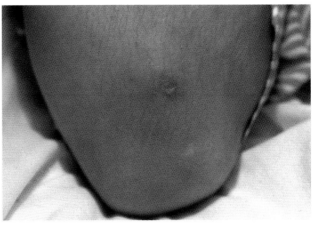

43-4. *Lesions are usually sparse and scattered over the extremities.*

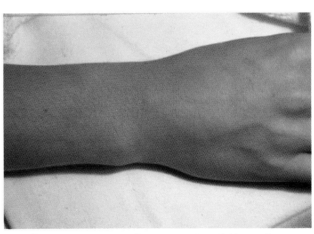

43-5. *Tenosynovitis is part of the dermatitis-arthritis syndrome.*

Petechiae, Purpura, or Ecchymoses

Infective endocarditis

Skin

Petechiae

- Lesions occur in 20% to 40% of cases. At first, lesions are red and nonblanching and commonly fade in two to three days. They usually appear in crops, especially in conjunctivae, buccal mucosa or palate, upper chest, and extremities. Rarely, numerous lesions occur on lower extremities.

Splinter hemorrhages

- Characteristic lesions are linear red-to-brown streaks under fingernails or toenails or both.

Osler's nodes

- These lesions, 2 to 15 mm in diameter, are erythematous, wheal-like, tender nodules usually located on pads of fingers and toes. They are frequently evanescent, lasting a few hours to days.

Janeway lesions

- Characteristic lesions are small, erythematous, painless macules or plaques or palpable purpura; they usually occur on the palms or soles.

Pathogenesis

- Infection of heart valves, with development of allergic (or immune complex) vasculitis or septic emboli, may be the cause.

Clinical features

- Symptoms and signs are protean and are more likely to be present in subacute than in acute endocarditis or early prosthetic valve endocarditis; fever (present in 95% of cases), chills, fatigue, malaise, anorexia, weight loss, arthralgias, myalgias, stroke, heart murmur (present in 85% of cases), splenomegaly, clubbing, and embolic phenomena may be present.

Differential diagnosis

- *Petechiae:* capillary angiomas, angiokeratomas.

- *Splinter hemorrhages:* trauma, foreign material, hypersensitivity vasculitis.

- *Osler's nodes or Janeway lesions:* hypersensitivity vasculitis, systemic lupus erythematosus, marantic endocarditis, hemolytic anemia, disseminated gonococcal infection.

Diagnostic tests

- Blood culture: Three cultures in first 24 hours yield etiologic diagnosis in up to 95% of cases; additional cultures may be needed in patients who have been receiving antibiotic therapy; if initial cultures are negative, consider causes of "culture-negative endocarditis."

Therapy

- High-dose microbicidal antibiotic therapy directed toward specific etiologic agent; therapy should be guided by antibiotic susceptibility testing (minimum inhibitory concentrations [MICs] and minimum bactericidal concentrations [MBCs]) and by serum bactericidal tests.

- In extremely ill patients, empiric therapy should be instituted before culture results are known.

- Decisions regarding surgery are guided by the specific etiologic agent, persistent or recurrent bacteremia, recurrent emboli, cardiac rhythm disturbance, or myocardial dysfunction.

Infective endocarditis

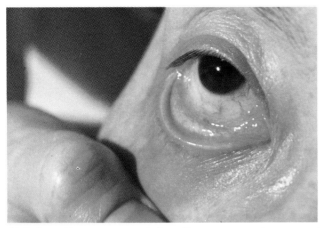

44-1. *Petechiae are commonly found in mucous membranes.*

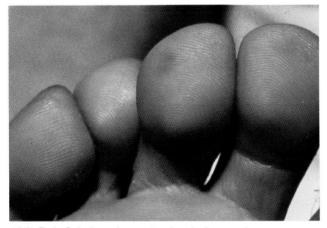

44-2. *Early Osler's nodes are tender, dusky macules.*

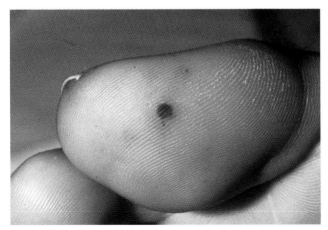

44-3. *Osler's nodes may later become more purpuric, necrotic, or pustular.*

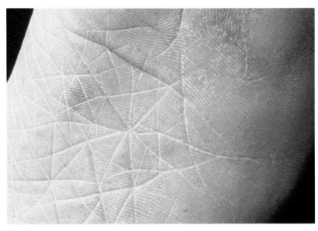

44-4. *Janeway lesions most commonly occur on the palms or soles and are painless.*

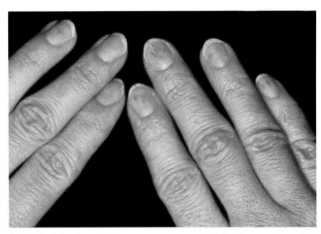

44-5. *Splinter hemorrhages are common in infective endocarditis but are not pathognomonic.*

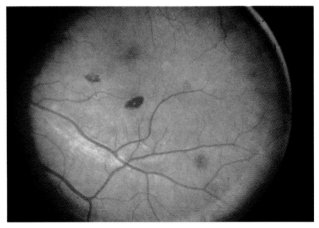

44-6. *These retinal hemorrhages of infective endocarditis are called Roth's spots.*

Petechiae, Purpura, or Ecchymoses

Dengue

Skin

Classic dengue fever

- Early transient rash appears on elbows and knees; from days two to five, a morbilliform or scarlatiniform rash appears on the chest and spreads centrifugally. During the last days of fever, petechiae appear on extremities, axillae, or mucous membranes (in 20% to 70% of cases).

Dengue hemorrhagic fever (DHF)

- Hemorrhagic manifestations—petechiae, purpura, or ecchymoses—may develop.

Pathogenesis

- Group B togavirus is transmitted to man by the *Aedes* mosquito.
- Small dermal blood vessel injury occurs in classic dengue fever.
- Diffuse hemorrhage into serous cavities, hepatic necrosis, disseminated intravascular coagulation, and complement activation occur in DHF.

Clinical features

- Persons who travel to or reside in epidemic areas (Caribbean, Pacific, Southeast Asia, and some areas of Mexico) are predisposed.
- *Classic dengue fever:* This is a benign illness with fever lasting five to seven days; accompanying symptoms may be severe headache, eye pain, conjunctival injection, backache, marked muscle and joint pain (breakbone fever), lymphadenopathy, fatigue, anorexia, and constipation.
- *DHF:* This disease usually affects children less than 14 years old. Occasionally adults are affected, and bleeding usually develops, without shock. Hemorrhagic shock syndrome (8% mortality) is characterized by vomiting, cyanosis, dyspnea, hepatomegaly, epistaxis, hematemesis, melena, and hypotension.

Differential diagnosis

- Rubella, rubeola, enteroviral or hepatitis virus infections, meningococcemia, rickettsial infections, typhoid fever, leptospirosis, scarlet fever.
- Allergic (drug-related) reactions.

Diagnostic tests

- Acute and convalescent serum for dengue virus antibody levels.
- Virus isolation.

Therapy

- *Classic dengue fever:* Symptomatic relief.
- *DHF:* Supportive care; possibly systemic steroids.

Dengue

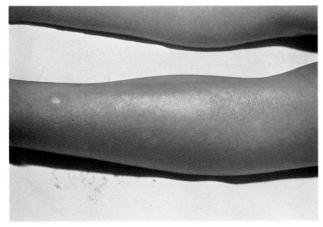

45-1. *In classic dengue fever, the early rash is often scarlatiniform. Note also the "white islands in a sea of red."*

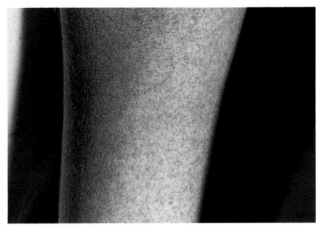

45-4. *A shower of petechiae occurred soon after a tourniquet was applied to this patient who had dengue hemorrhagic fever.*

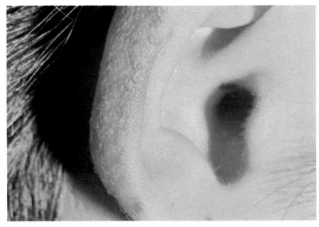

45-2. *In dengue hemorrhagic fever, scattered areas of purpura may be present.*

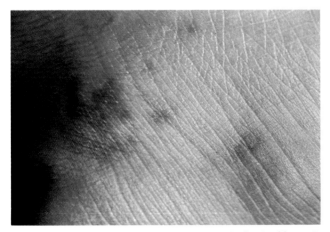

45-3. *Purpura on palms and soles may mimic Rocky Mountain spotted fever.*

Petechiae, Purpura, or Ecchymoses

Plague

Skin

- Petechiae and erythematous papules (often pruritic) are most common. Rarely, vesicles, bullae, or umbilicated pustules develop, with a predilection for the trunk.
- Purpura and ecchymoses may develop, especially in septicemic plague.
- A small papule or vesicopustule is seen occasionally at the site of the flea bite.
- Cutaneous lesions occur in only about 10% of cases.

Pathogenesis

- *Yersinia pestis,* a gram-negative bacillus, with safety-pin bipolar staining, maintained in a rodent-flea infection cycle, accidentally infects humans. In the United States, infection is commonly initiated by contact with rodents (rock or ground squirrels, prairie dogs, and wood rats) or lagomorphs (rabbits and hares).
- Pyogenic, necrotic, infarctive, hemorrhagic damage of multiple organ systems occurs—especially the lymphatics, liver, spleen, lungs, mucous membranes, and meninges.
- Endotoxemia, Shwartzman-like reactions, and disseminated intravascular coagulopathy play roles in pathogenesis.
- Primary pneumonic plague results from direct inhalation of organisms.

Clinical features

- Persons who travel to or reside in an endemic area (such as New Mexico and California) are predisposed.
- Buboes: Painful, tender, enlarged lymph nodes are observed in bubonic plague. (Inguinal and axillary adenitis and periadenitis are most common.)
- In early infections, detectable lymphadenopathy may not be present or may never develop (primary septicemic plague).
- Fever, chills, headache, myalgias, arthralgias, and cough are common.
- Shock, bleeding diathesis, and congestive heart failure may develop.
- Fulminant pneumonia occurs in primary pneumonic plague.

Differential diagnosis

- Painful, tender lymphadenopathy and systemic symptoms: tularemia, staphylococcal or streptococcal suppurative lymphadenopathy, lymphogranuloma venereum, cat-scratch disease.
- Septicemic plague: meningococcemia, gram-negative bacteremia, disseminated intravascular coagulopathy, Rocky Mountain spotted fever.

Diagnostic tests

- Gram stain or special fluorescent antibody staining of aspirates from a bubo or parabubo tissue, purulent drainage, or sputum.
- Blood cultures (four cultures over one to two hours).
- Needle aspirate of bubo for culture (organisms grow relatively slowly).
- Acute and convalescent sera for *Y pestis* antibody levels.

Therapy

- Strict isolation of all patients.
- Antibiotics (streptomycin and tetracycline) initiated rapidly, before diagnosis established.
- Supportive care.

Plague

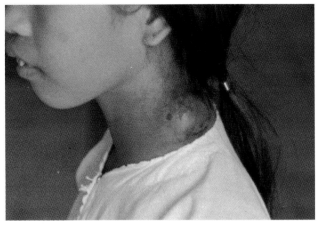

46-1. *Buboes are painful, tender, enlarged lymph nodes.*

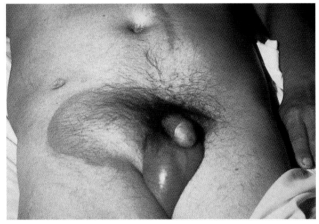

46-2. *The overlying skin of this bubo was cleaned with iodine prior to aspiration.*

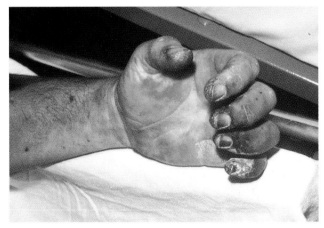

46-3. *In septicemic plague, purpura, ecchymosis, or even frank gangrene may develop.*

Ulcers or Necrosis

Genital Ulcers*

Disease	Etiology	Lesions	Lympha-denopathy	Systemic symptoms	Diagnostic tests	Therapy
Primary syphilis	· *Treponema pallidum.*	· A painless papule progresses to an ulcer (chancre). · Smooth base. · Raised, firm border. · Painless. · Usually singular.	· Regional, non-tender, rubbery, nonsuppurative bilateral lymph-adenopathy occurs three to four days after chancre appears.	· None.	· Dark-field examination. · FTA-ABS** (positive in 85% of cases). · VDRL** (positive in 70% of cases).	· Penicillin.
Genital herpes	· Herpes simplex virus.	· Painful vesicles occur on erythe-matous base. · Usually multiple.	· In primary infec-tion, tender, bi-lateral inguinal adenopathy develops.	· Present during primary infection.	· Multinucleated giant cells (stained smear of vesicle base). · Culture.	· Symptomatic.
Chancroid	· *Hemophilus ducreyi.*	· A tender papule progresses to a pustule, then to a painful, nonindu-rated ulcer. · Ragged edges. · Single or multiple.	· Tender, regional, painful, sup-purative nodes develop.	· None.	· Gram stain. · Culture.	· Sulfonamide.
Lympho-granuloma venereum	· *Chlamydia trachomatis.*	· A small painless vesicle or papule progresses to an ulcer. · Heals quickly.	· Painful, matted, necrotic, fluc-tuant, large nodes develop, with fistula tracts (after genital lesion heals).	· Present after genital lesion heals.	· CF** or IF** anti-body titers (cul-tures positive in 30% of cases).	· Sulfonamide.
Granuloma inguinale (Donovanosis)	· *Calymmato-bacterium granulomatis.*	· A painless, indu-rated nodule progresses to a beefy, exuberant, heaped-up ulcer.	· Pseudobuboes.	· None.	· Donovan bodies (stain crushed tissue).	· Tetracycline.

*Diseases listed are usually sexually transmitted. Differential diagnosis of genital ulcers should include: Behcet's syndrome, erythema multiforme, traumatic lesions, and carcinoma.
**FTA-ABS: Fluorescent treponemal antibody-absorption test for syphilis
VDRL: Veneral Disease Research Laboratories
CF: Complement fixation
IF: Indirect fluorescence

Genital ulcers

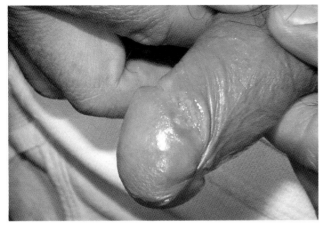

47-1. *The chancre of primary syphilis is a painless, indurated, solitary ulcer.*

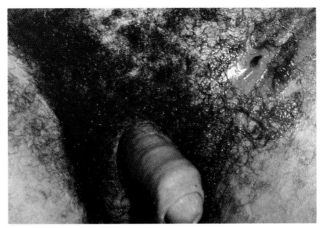

47-4. *The genital ulcer of lymphogranuloma venereum is usually not seen. Painful, suppurating inguinal lymph nodes may be the presenting symptom.*

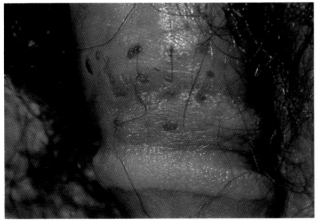

47-2. *Multiple painful grouped ulcerations suggest genital herpes.*

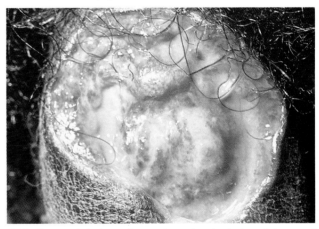

47-5. *The genital ulcer of granuloma inguinale is painless and heaped up with granulation tissue.*

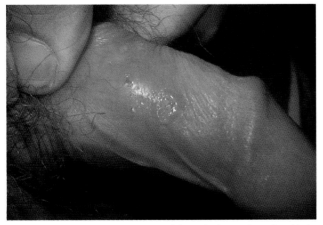

47-3. *Ulcers of chancroid are painful, nonindurated, and multiple, with ragged edges.*

Ulcers or Necrosis

Impetigo

Skin

- Primary lesions are small vesicles that rupture quickly to form purulent erosions, often covered with characteristic honey-colored, stuck-on, thick crusts.

- One or many lesions may be present.

- Lesions are usually painless but may itch, burn, or sting.

- In bullous impetigo, flaccid bullae are filled with pus, which may layer out.

Pathogenesis

- Impetigo is a skin infection caused by group A streptococci (rarely groups B, C, or G), although *Staphylococcus aureus* may also be isolated.

- It may occur at sites of eczema, arthropod bites, varicella, traumatic erosions, or places where the epidermal barrier is lacking.

- Bullous impetigo is caused by *S aureus*, phage group II.

- Impetigo is highly communicable to other body sites (autoinoculation) or other persons.

Clinical features

- Mainly, children are affected.

- Infection is usually limited to the skin.

- Lymphadenopathy and leukocytosis may be present.

- Glomerulonephritis rarely occurs.

Differential diagnosis

- Herpes simplex virus infection, varicella, pemphigus, traumatic erosion, acute dermatitis, bites.

Diagnostic tests

- Usually a clinical diagnosis.

- Gram stain or culture.

- AntiDNase B and streptococcal hyaluronidase titers usually rise after infection, but the antistreptolysin-O (ASO) titer often does not.

Therapy

- Systemic penicillin G or equivalent or erythromycin for ten days.

- Antistaphylococcal antibiotic for bullous impetigo.

- Compresses or soaks twice a day to remove crusts.

- Topical antibiotic ointments only as adjuncts to systemic antibiotics.

Impetigo

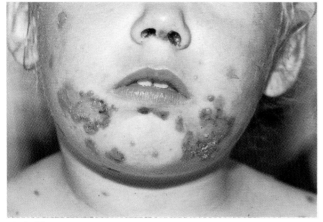

48-1. *Weeping or crusted erosions are characteristic.*

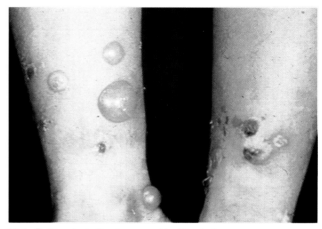

48-4. *Bullous impetigo is caused by Staphylococcus aureus.*

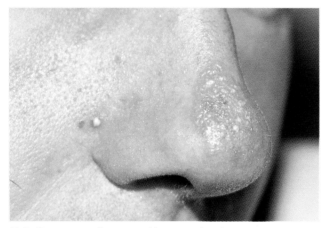

48-2. *Crusts are adherent and honey-colored.*

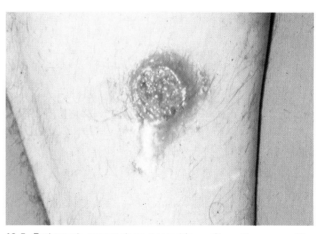

48-5. *Ecthyma is a more deep-seated form of impetigo caused by group A streptococci.*

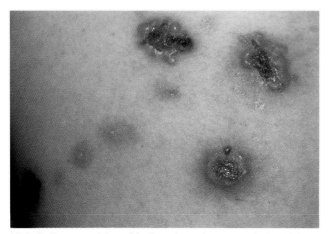

48-3. *Delicate vesicles of bullous impetigo may mimic chicken-pox.*

Ulcers or Necrosis

Ecthyma gangrenosum

Skin
- Lesions begin as painful red macules that enlarge and become slightly elevated papules.
- Hemorrhage and necrosis are characteristic.
- Older lesions are ulcers usually with hemorrhagic crust or eschar.
- Lesions are characterized by a central area of purple-to-black necrosis, with sharply defined geographic margins.
- A single lesion may be present, but usually multiple lesions of various stages are seen.
- Lesions appear most frequently on the lower trunk and extremities.

Pathogenesis
- Lesions are most commonly associated with *Pseudomonas aeruginosa* bacteremia but are not always caused by this agent. (Other gram-negative bacterial etiologies include *Aeromonas, Proteus, E coli, Enterobacter,* and *Klebsiella;* rarely, *Candida* is the cause.)
- Bacteria invade the vein wall; fibrin thrombi cause occlusion of small vessels, which in turn causes infarction and necrosis.

Clinical features
- The patient is usually immunocompromised, often neutropenic.
- Symptoms and signs of gram-negative bacteremia are present.

Differential diagnosis
- Cutaneous vasculitis, hypersensitivity angiitis, suppurating panniculitis, necrotizing cellulitis (see section titled Necrotizing [Gangrenous] Cellulitis), gonococcemia, pyoderma gangrenosum.

Diagnostic tests
- Biopsy or scrapings from base of lesion may reveal gram-negative bacilli (Gram stain and culture).

Therapy
- Systemic antibiotics.
- Supportive care.
- Prolonged soaks to debride crusts and necrotic debris.

Ecthyma gangrenosum

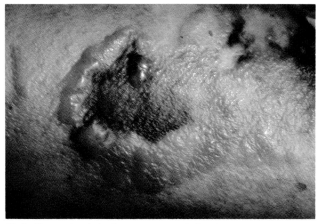

49-1. *Hemorrhagic bullae may precede frank necrosis.*

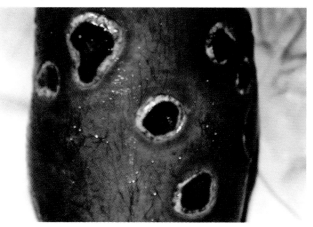

49-4. *Pseudomonas aeruginosa is the most common cause of ecthyma gangrenosum.*

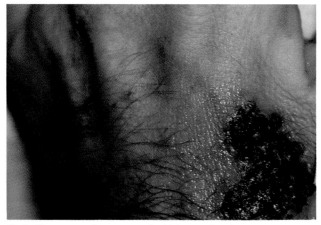

49-2. *Ulcers are often covered with hemorrhagic crusts.*

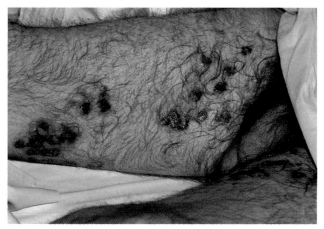

49-3. *Lower extremities are frequently involved, and multiple lesions are common.*

Ulcers or Necrosis

Sporotrichosis

Skin

Lymphocutaneous sporotrichosis

• The most common and classic manifestation of sporotrichosis, this infection appears initially as a painless pink, purple, or black papule, usually on the hand, where it enlarges slowly and ulcerates. Subsequently, multiple, painless, red-to-violet ulcerated nodules develop along lymphatic channels that drain the initial lesion. Interconnecting lymphatics may be palpable. Lesions rarely spread to cause disseminated cutaneous involvement. Extremities are most commonly involved in adults, and the face and trunk are more commonly involved in children.

Cutaneous sporotrichosis or fixed or plaque sporotrichosis

• These variations account for 20% to 30% of cases of sporotrichosis. No lymphatic involvement accompanies these painless ulcerated nodules, verrucous nodules, or nonspecific erythematous plaques. Lesions most commonly appear on the trunk, face, or neck.

Focal or multifocal (systemic) extracutaneous sporotrichosis

• Numerous dusky-red nodules scattered over the body enlarge up to several centimeters and produce ulceration and suppuration. Cutaneous lesions may be absent, especially in focal sporotrichosis.

Pathogenesis

• *Lymphocutaneous or cutaneous sporotrichosis* results when the fungus *Sporothrix schenckii* is inoculated into the skin by trauma; lesions occur seven days to six months later and are only rarely followed by systemic disease.

• *Extracutaneous sporotrichosis* results from focal inoculation into the skin or from hematogenous dissemination of *S schenckii* from a primary pulmonary focus; compromised host defenses may predispose a person to systemic disease.

• Dense granulomatous response with microabscesses may result.

Clinical features

• Persons exposed to soil (gardeners, farmers, florists) are at greatest risk.

• In lymphocutaneous and cutaneous infections, no constitutional symptoms or signs develop unless lesions become secondarily infected with bacteria.

• Focal and multifocal extracutaneous infections involve a variety of sites, including the osteoarticular, pulmonary, and central nervous systems.

Differential diagnosis

• *Lymphocutaneous sporotrichosis*: atypical mycobacterial infection (especially *M marinum*), primary cutaneous nocardiosis, cutaneous leishmaniasis.

• *Cutaneous sporotrichosis*: chromomycosis, blastomycosis, coccidioidomycosis, cryptococcosis, tuberculosis verrucosa cutis, verruca vulgaris, syphilitic chancre, leishmanial ulcer.

• *Extracutaneous sporotrichosis*: mimics a variety of more common diseases.

Diagnostic tests

• Culture tissue (by biopsy) or pus (by aspiration) using Sabouraud's agar.

• Gomori's methenamine silver or periodic acid-Schiff (PAS) stains of tissue to detect oval or cigar-shaped yeasts.

Therapy

• *Lymphocutaneous or cutaneous sporotrichosis*: potassium iodide orally, heat locally.

• *Extracutaneous sporotrichosis*: amphotericin B intravenously.

Sporotrichosis

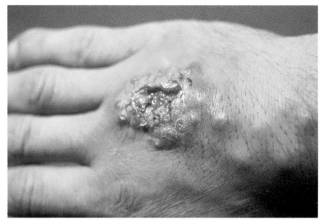

50-1. *The typical lesion is an ulcerated, violaceous nodule.*

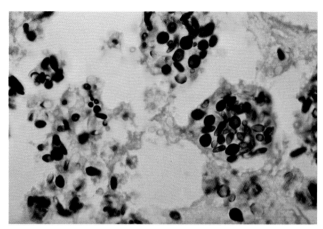

50-4. *Cigar-shaped yeasts are sometimes seen in tissue stained with Gomori's methenamine silver.*

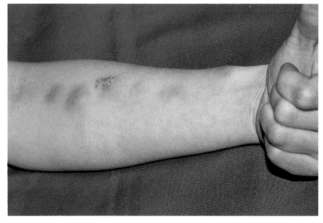

50-2. *Multiple red nodules develop along draining lymphatic channels in lymphocutaneous sporotrichosis.*

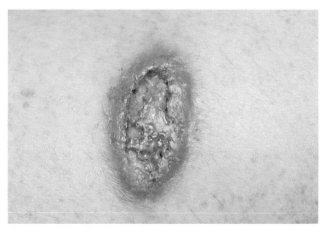

50-3. *In the fixed form, there is no lymphatic involvement.*

Ulcers or Necrosis

Atypical mycobacteria

Skin
- Characteristics are variable, depending on the organism involved.
- An undermined, enlarging, painless ulcer may be present.
- A papule is often present at a site of trauma, usually on the hands, elbows, feet, or knees. The papule progresses to a nodule or plaque that often ulcerates.
- Sporotrichoid spread with satellite lesions along regional lymphatics may occur.
- Suppurative cervical adenitis or skin abscesses may develop.

Pathogenesis
- The skin is infected by *Mycobacterium marinum* (swimming pool granuloma), *M ulcerans* (Buruli ulcer), *M scrofulaceum* (scrofuloderma), *M kansasii, M chelonei, M intracellulare,* or other atypical mycobacteria.
- Inoculation of the skin rarely results in hematogenous dissemination.
- *M marinum* (most common in the United States) is present in some swimming pools and fish tanks as well as fresh and salt water.

Clinical features
- Findings are variable, depending on the organism involved; usually systemic infection does not occur.
- *M kansasii* and *M intracellulare* may cause pulmonary infections that simulate tuberculosis, osteomyelitis, and lymphadenitis.

Differential diagnosis
- Sporotrichosis, tuberculosis verrucosa cutis, coccidioidomycosis, blastomycosis, histoplasmosis, syphilitic gumma, tularemia, nocardiosis, tuberculous scrofuloderma, ulcerating carcinoma, verruca vulgaris.

Diagnostic tests
- Biopsy with Fite or other stain to detect acid-fast bacteria.
- Culture—usually at 32°C and 37°C.
- Intradermal skin tests: purified protein derivative (PPD) test, and if available, PPD tests of various atypical mycobacteria.

Therapy
- Often self-healing within two years.
- Excision.
- Antituberculous drugs, guided by sensitivity tests.

Atypical mycobacteria

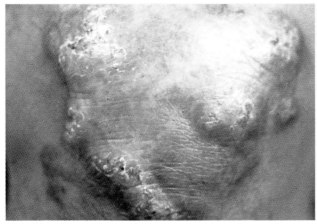

51-1. Mycobacterium marinum commonly produces ulcerated nodules on the knee, elbow, foot, or hand.

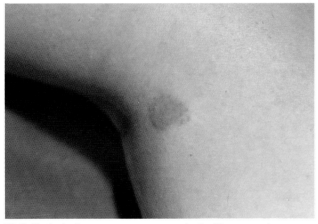

51-2. Early lesions may appear as insignificant erythematous plaques.

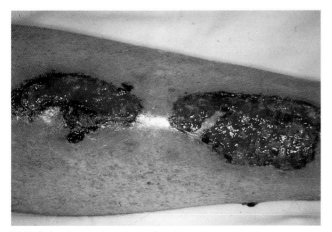

51-3. Later, large ulcers may develop.

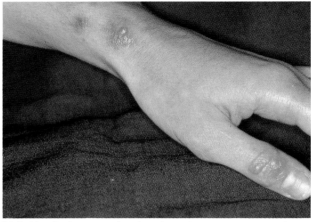

51-4. New lesions may develop along draining lymphatics (sporotrichoid spread).

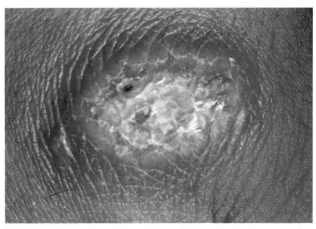

51-5. An ulcerated nodule with a rolled, raised edge may be mistaken for carcinoma.

Ulcers or Necrosis

Nocardiosis

Skin

Primary cutaneous nocardiosis

• This infection produces a variety of lesions, including cellulitis, pustules, abscesses, and the ulcerated nodules (chancriform) of lymphocutaneous sporotrichoid syndrome (mimics cutaneous sporotrichosis—see section titled Sporotrichosis).

Mycetoma (madura foot)

• This infection begins as papules and nodules that slowly progress to produce indurated skin and soft-tissue swelling, with multiple sinus tracts draining granule-filled pus; most commonly, the foot or hand is involved.

Secondary cutaneous nocardiosis

• This infection is manifest as single or multiple firm subcutaneous abscesses.

Pathogenesis

• *Primary cutaneous nocardiosis* is caused by traumatic introduction of *Nocardia sp (N brasiliensis* more often than *N asteroides)* into the skin from soil; host defenses are usually normal.

• *Mycetoma* is caused by traumatic introduction of one species of a variety of either true fungi or actinomycetes, including *N brasiliensis, N asteroides,* and *N caviae,* into the skin from soil; host defenses are usually normal. Infection eventually involves subcutaneous tissues, muscle, and bone.

• *Secondary cutaneous nocardiosis* is caused by hematogenous dissemination, usually from a pulmonary focus, of *Nocardia (N asteroides* more often than *N brasiliensis)*; host defenses are usually compromised.

Clinical features

• *In primary cutaneous nocardiosis and mycetoma,* findings are usually local. (There is rarely dissemination to internal organs.)

• *In secondary cutaneous nocardiosis,* concomitant pulmonary infection or central nervous system infection or both are usually present.

Differential diagnosis

• *Primary cutaneous nocardiosis:* skin infection due to *Staphylococcus aureus,* atypical mycobacteria, *Sporothrix schenckii.*

• *Mycetoma:* skin, soft-tissue, or bone infection due to organisms such as *Allescheria boydii,* other deep tissue fungi, *S aureus,* elephantiasis, tuberculosis.

• *Secondary cutaneous nocardiosis:* subcutaneous abscesses due to a variety of opportunistic organisms, actinomycosis, tuberculosis, syphilis, granuloma inguinale, furunculosis.

Diagnostic tests

• Gram stain (delicate, weakly gram-positive, beaded, branching filaments).

• Modified acid-fast bacterial stain (organisms are weakly acid fast).

• Culture (aerobic—blood or chocolate agar): organisms grow slowly (hold culture for longer than one week); madura foot—deep-tissue biopsy material cultured on Sabouraud's medium, without antibiotics added.

• Sulfur granules (colonies of organisms) seen commonly in mycetoma but rarely seen in primary cutaneous nocardiosis (sulfur granules also seen in other diseases, including actinomycosis and *S aureus* infections).

Therapy

• *Primary cutaneous nocardiosis:* drainage of abscesses, short course of sulfonamide therapy.

• *Mycetoma* (due to *Nocardia*): long-term sulfonamide or trimethoprim-sulfamethoxazole therapy.

• *Secondary cutaneous nocardiosis:* long-term sulfonamide therapy.

Nocardiosis

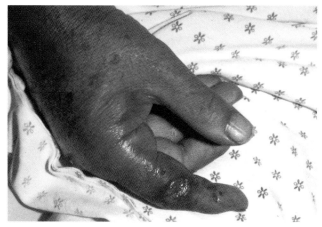

52-1. *Nocardia brasiliensis infection occurred following trauma suffered by this gardener.*

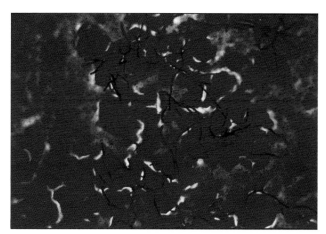

52-4. *Nocardia is a filamentous, aerobic, gram-positive bacterium.*

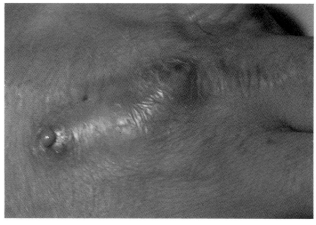

52-2. *Cutaneous nocardiosis may cause draining sinuses.*

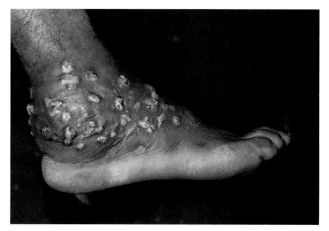

52-3. *Nocardia is only one of many infectious agents that cause madura foot.*

Ulcers or Necrosis

Histoplasmosis

Skin

Disseminated histoplasmosis

• This infection is accompanied by ulcerated or indurated plaques in the mouth, especially the soft palate, in about 20% of patients. Skin lesions are rare and of variable morphology; most characteristic lesions are painless, punched-out ulcers. Less commonly, papules, plaques, pustules, vesicles, and purpura develop. Complications include erythema nodosum, erythema multiforme, and exfoliative erythroderma.

Primary cutaneous histoplasmosis

• This infection is extremely rare. A tender, erythematous nodule or ulcer (chancriform syndrome) is accompanied by lymphangitis and regional lymphadenopathy.

Pathogenesis

• *Disseminated histoplasmosis* is caused by hematogenous dissemination of the fungus *Histoplasma capsulatum* from a pulmonary focus to mucous membranes or skin. Lesions often occur in patients who have compromised host defenses and may represent reactivation of fungus many years after primary pulmonary infection occurred.

• *Primary cutaneous histoplasmosis* is caused by inoculation of *H capsulatum* into the skin, with lesion development at the entry site.

Clinical features

• *Disseminated histoplasmosis:* clinical evidence of systemic disease is variable and may involve the lungs, meninges, liver, spleen, bone marrow, and adrenals.

• *Primary cutaneous histoplasmosis:* history of occupational exposure is helpful; findings are limited to the skin.

Differential diagnosis

• Mucous membranes: Wegner's granulomatosis, carcinoma, lethal midline granuloma, mucormycosis.

• Skin (ulcerative lesions): atypical mycobacterial infection, sporotrichosis, primary syphilis, nocardiosis.

Diagnostic tests

• Tissue biopsy (of skin, bone marrow, liver, or lung) for methenamine silver and periodic acid-Schiff (PAS) stains and for culture (Sabouraud's agar); organism grows slowly (two to four weeks for positive culture).

• Serologic tests and skin test are not helpful.

Therapy

• *Disseminated histoplasmosis:* amphotericin B intravenously.

• *Primary cutaneous histoplasmosis:* heals spontaneously.

Histoplasmosis

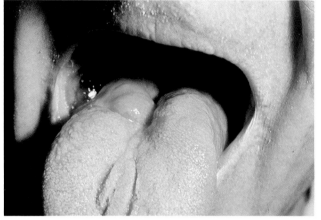

53-1. *Mucous membranes are involved more commonly than is skin.*

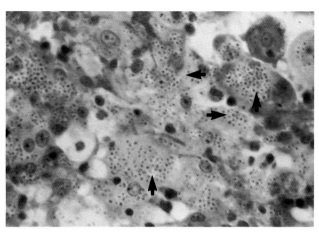

53-4. *Numerous small yeast cells are present in macrophages.*

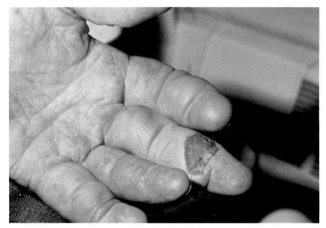

53-2. *The most characteristic lesion of cutaneous histoplasmosis is a punched-out ulcer.*

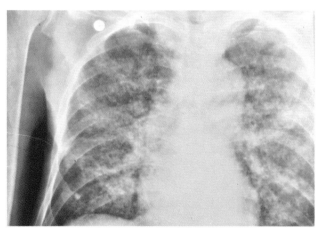

53-5. *Evidence of disseminated histoplasmosis is seen in this patient's chest x-ray film.*

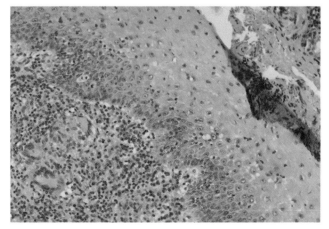

53-3. *Biopsy of cutaneous histoplasmosis shows a granulomatous infiltrate with multinucleated giant cells.*

Ulcers or Necrosis

Anthrax

Skin
• Infection begins as an erythematous macule or painless papule, which enlarges and becomes a pruritic vesicle or bulla (containing clear-to-dark fluid) that progresses to a hemorrhagic necrotic ulcer covered by a black crust (malignant pustule) on a gelatinous, brawny, edematous base.

• It most commonly occurs on the face, neck, or arms.

• It heals with a scar.

Pathogenesis
• *Bacillus anthracis* spores enter a break in the skin, germinate, multiply, and produce a toxin; infection may disseminate via the bloodstream.

Clinical features
• Often there is a history of exposure to contaminated imported wool, hides, or bone meal.

• Inoculation anthrax is most commonly limited to the skin.

• Patient may have low-grade fever and malaise.

• Bacteremic dissemination from the skin may be associated with high fever, hypotension, and meningitis.

Differential diagnosis
• Staphylococcal furuncle or abscess, tularemia, plague, milker's nodules, orf, cellulitis, cutaneous diphtheria.

Diagnostic tests
• Gram stain and culture (routine media) of vesicular fluid or fluid beneath crust.

Therapy
• Systemic penicillin.

• Severe cases: supportive care.

• Incision and debridement *not* recommended.

Anthrax

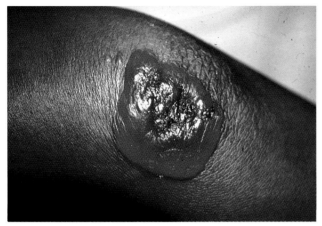

54-1. *The malignant pustule of anthrax is a necrotic ulcer on a gelatinous, edematous base.*

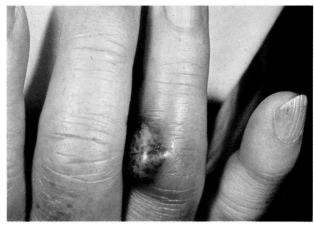

54-4. *Cutaneous diphtheria is occasionally mistaken for anthrax.*

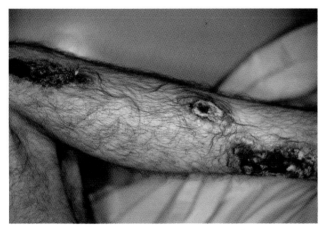

54-2. *In later stages, ulcers are covered with eschar.*

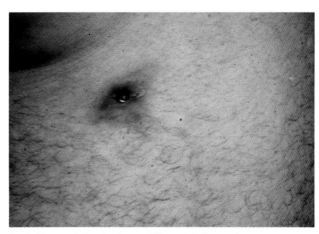

54-5. *Tularemia is also in the differential diagnosis.*

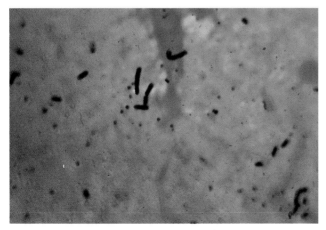

54-3. *Bacillus anthracis is a gram-positive bacterium.*

Nail Infections

Onychomycosis

Nails
- A brown discoloration appears at the distal edge of the nails.
- Nails become soft, thick, and irregular, and they separate from the nail bed.
- Scales of skin seem to collect under the nail plate and lift the distal end.
- Usually more than one nail is involved (often all toe nails).
- The superficial white type is characterized by a white discoloration on the top of the nail, near the proximal nail fold, but the nail is not dystrophic.

Skin
- Often, there is coexisting chronic tinea pedis, which usually appears as a noninflammatory, dust-like scaling in moccasin distribution, bilaterally.
  Recurrent symptomatic interdigital fissures (athlete's foot) are also common.

Pathogenesis
- Infection of the nail plate with *Trichophyton rubrum, T mentagrophytes,* or rarely other *Trichophyton* species; *Candida albicans* and *Scopulariopsis brevicaulis* are other causes.

Clinical features
- Infection is limited to the skin and nails.

Differential diagnosis
- Psoriasis, onychodystrophy of other causes, Darier's disease, lichen planus, dermatitis of skin adjacent to nails.

Diagnostic tests
- Potassium hydroxide (KOH) examination of subungual debris.
- Superficial white type: KOH examination of scrapings from the white portion of the nail itself.
- Culture (Sabouraud's with antibacterials).

Therapy
- Clotrimazole, haloprogin, or miconazole solution applied topically.
- Surgical or medical avulsion.
- Systemic griseofulvin for six months to one year.

Onychomycosis

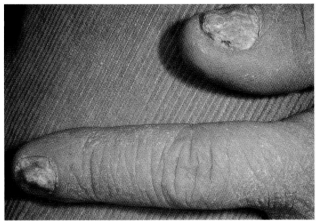

55-1. *Fungal infection of the nails frequently is associated with fungal infection of the adjacent skin.*

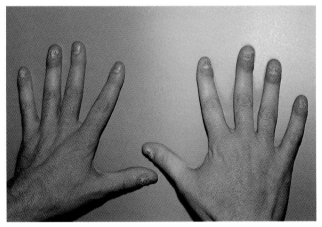

55-2. *Patients who have mucocutaneous candidiasis have chronic candidal infections of the nails.*

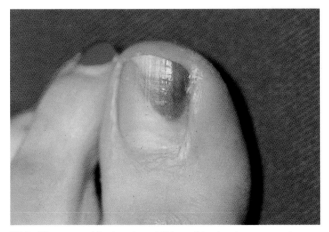

55-3. *The green-black color of this nail is due to pyocyanin produced by Pseudomonas aeruginosa.*

Credits

Figures 2-1, 2-3, 2-4, and 2-5 are reprinted with permission from Caroline B. Hall, MD, University of Rochester Medical Center, Rochester, New York, and *Annals of Internal Medicine* 90:882-886, 1979.

Figures 5-5, 12-1, 22-2, 24-2, 24-3, 27-4, 34-3, 36-2, 36-3, 37-1, 48-4, and 48-5 are reprinted with permission from Samuel M. Bluefarb, MD, Northwestern University Medical School, Chicago, Illinois.

Figures 9-4 and 53-4 are reprinted with permission from Glenn S. Bulmer, PhD, The University of Oklahoma Medical Center, Oklahoma City, Oklahoma.

Figures 15-2, 23-1, 23-4, 26-1, 26-5, and 28-1 are reprinted with permission from Mark V. Dahl, MD, and *Modern Medicine* 45:42-46, 1977; 46:48-60, 1979; 47:82-85, 1978; 48:38-46, 1980.

Figure 20-3 is reprinted with permission from Sydney M. Finegold, MD, Veterans Administration, Wadsworth Hospital, Los Angeles, California, and Martin McHenry, MD, Cleveland Clinic, Cleveland, Ohio.

Figures 21-2 and 21-3 are reprinted with permission from Sydney M. Finegold, MD, Veterans Administration, Wadsworth Hospital, Los Angeles, California, and James Taylor, MD, Long Beach Veterans Administration Hospital, Long Beach, California.

Figures 41-1, 41-2, 41-3, 41-4, and 41-5 are reprinted with permission from David Durack, MD, Duke University Medical Center, Durham, North Carolina, and Merle Sande, MD, San Francisco General Hospital, San Francisco, California.

Figures 44-1, 44-2, 44-3, 44-5, and 44-6 are reprinted with permission from Paul E. Hermans, MD, Mayo Clinic, Rochester, Minnesota, and *Mayo Clinic Proceedings* 57:15-21, 1982.

Figures 45-1, 45-2, 45-3, and 45-4 are reprinted with permission from Robert McNair Scott III, MD, Walter Reed Army Institute of Research, Walter Reed Army Medical Center, Washington, DC.

Figure 46-3 is reprinted with permission from the Centers for Disease Control, Atlanta, Georgia.

Index

Index